WRITING SKILLS IN NURSING AND HEALTHCARE

WRITING SKILLS IN NURSING AND HEALTHCARE

A GUIDE TO COMPLETING SUCCESSFUL DISSERTATIONS AND THESES

DENA BAIN TAYLOR

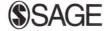
SAGE

Los Angeles | London | New Delhi
Singapore | Washington DC

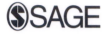

Los Angeles | London | New Delhi
Singapore | Washington DC

SAGE Publications Ltd
1 Oliver's Yard
55 City Road
London EC1Y 1SP

SAGE Publications Inc.
2455 Teller Road
Thousand Oaks, California 91320

SAGE Publications India Pvt Ltd
B 1/I 1 Mohan Cooperative Industrial Area
Mathura Road
New Delhi 110 044

SAGE Publications Asia-Pacific Pte Ltd
3 Church Street
#10-04 Samsung Hub
Singapore 049483

Editor: Kate Wharton
Editorial Assistant: Laura Walmsley
Production editor: Katie Forsythe
Copyeditor: Clare Weaver
Proofreader: Christine Bitten
Marketing manager: Camille Richmond
Cover design: Naomi Robinson
Typeset by: C&M Digitals (P) Ltd, Chennai, India
Printed in India at Replika Press Pvt Ltd

© Dena Bain Taylor 2014

First published 2014

Library of Congress Control Number: 2013950721

British Library Cataloguing in Publication data

A catalogue record for this book is available from
the British Library

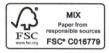

MIX
Paper from
responsible sources
FSC
www.fsc.org **FSC® C016779**

ISBN 978-1-4462-4746-4
ISBN 978-1-4462-4747-1 (pbk)

At SAGE we take sustainability seriously. Most of our products are printed in the UK using FSC papers and boards.
When we print overseas we ensure sustainable papers are used as measured by the Egmont grading system.
We undertake an annual audit to monitor our sustainability.

TABLE OF CONTENTS

ABOUT THE AUTHOR

Dena Bain Taylor holds a PhD in English from the University of Toronto, Canada, where she has taught since 1985. As Director of the Health Sciences Writing Centre, she has 19 years of interdisciplinary experience teaching writing and critical skills across the full range of health professions, most notably with undergraduate and graduate students in the Lawrence S. Bloomberg Faculty of Nursing, Canada's largest school of Nursing. In 2012 she was awarded the University of Toronto's prestigious Joan E. Foley Award for Quality of Student Experience. Her academic publications include *Writing Skills for Nursing and Midwifery Students* (2013), the *Young Learner's Illustrated English-Chinese Dictionary* (1994) and the online *Writing in the Health Sciences: A Comprehensive Guide* (2008). She lives in a small palace in the sky overlooking Lake Ontario.

ACKNOWLEDGEMENTS

The author and publishers would like to thank those who have provided example dissertations for inclusion in this book.

Karen Eisler, RN, BScN, MScN, PhD, Executive Director, Saskatchewan Registered Nurses' Association, Regina, Saskatchewan.

Jennifer Lapum, RN, PhD, Associate Professor, Daphne Cockwell School of Nursing, Ryerson University, Toronto, Ontario.

Sarah Jane McGeorge, RGN, RMN, BSc (Hons), DProf; Nurse Consultant and Clinical Director at Tees, Esk and Wear Valleys NHS Foundation Trust, UK.

Stephen Moore, PhD, Professor of Healthcare Policy, Faculty of Medical Sciences, Anglia Ruskin University, Cambridge, UK.

Munikumar Ramasamy Venkatasalu, RGN, RMN, RNT, PhD, Senior Lecturer in Adult Nursing, Faculty of Health & Social Sciences, Bedfordshire University, Aylesbury, UK.

Faith Wight Moffatt, RN, PhD, Assistant Professor, School of Nursing, Dalhousie University, Halifax, Nova Scotia.

1

INTRODUCTION TO THE POST-GRADUATE STUDENT EXPERIENCE

ABOUT THIS BOOK

The complex environment of contemporary healthcare places high value on evidence-based practice and multidisciplinary team approaches. One result is an emphasis on engaging in education throughout one's career. This has contributed, over approximately the past 20 years, to a worldwide explosion of enrolments in post-graduate and post-registration programmes in Nursing and allied health professions. Another major factor is the aging of the population in the developed world at a time of nursing shortages, which are themselves the result of complex factors. Schools of Nursing have responded by increasing enrolments to train new nurses; this, and a variety of workplace and policy contexts, have created a need for more Masters- and doctorate-trained professionals and lecturers. Finally, as the knowledge base produced by Nursing and allied health research grows in breadth and stature, there is an ever-increasing need to train researchers in both academic and professional settings, both Masters and PhD prepared.

Registered nurses, midwives and other health professionals enter post-graduate school programmes for a wide variety of reasons and only you can say why you are taking a post-graduate or post-registration degree (though we will talk a little later about the importance of keeping your expectations realistic). But there is no question that a post-registration degree can advance your career in a wide variety of directions. Whether you are interested in pursuing opportunities in advanced practice, management and administration, research, teaching, community health or any combination of these fields, a course of post-graduate study will help you develop advanced skills as a leader and practitioner.

Following the National Health Service's invaluable *Nursing Career Framework* and the Canadian Nurses Association's (2008) *Advanced Nursing Practice: A national framework*, this book approaches post-graduate writing within and across the following roles: research, teaching, leadership, management, and clinical. In this way, I hope you will find this book relevant no matter what role you hope to undertake in your career.

Although a book, of necessity, moves in a linear fashion from one topic to another, in reality, the post-graduate student experience encompasses numerous writing activities at the same time. For example, knowing that you have a deadline to submit a conference proposal, or a meeting scheduled with a supervisor, pushes you to write a portion of your thesis. Even the parts of being a student that interfere with your ability to write – for example, if you are also teaching or working – help to push you forward by giving you deadlines to write towards. As you careen down the road towards your degree, you may veer from one side to another, but you are always moving forward to your goal.

I intend this book as a resource on writing that can be used from the start of a post-registration Masters in Nursing or allied health professions through to the end of the doctoral degree programme. In writing it, I have kept in mind that students are often returning to an academic environment after years in practice and thus face added challenges in meeting the expectations of post-graduate studies, especially around academic writing.

The essential audience for this book is students in thesis-based programmes at the Masters or doctoral level. It will be much less relevant for students enrolled in a purely course-based Masters. For these students, there is a great deal of good advice on writing for courses in *Writing Skills for Nursing and Midwifery Students* (Taylor, 2013).

FOR FURTHER READING

Taylor, D.B. (2013) *Writing Skills for Nursing and Midwifery Students*. London: Sage Publications.

Canadian Nurses Association (2008) *Advanced Nursing Practice: A national framework*. Ottawa, ON: Author. Available at www2.cna-aiic.ca/CNA/documents/pdf/publications/ANP_National_Framework_e.pdf

National Health Service (nd) NHS Career Planner for Nurses. Available at http://nursingcareers.nhsemployers.org/

The dissertation models used in this book

A piece of advice given almost universally to students embarking on thesis writing is to look at previous dissertations from the department or on the internet. (The technical term at the doctoral level is 'dissertation' but most people simply say 'thesis'. Be prepared to respond to 'dissertation', however, especially if that is the term one of your examiners uses!) The advice is often couched in rather general terms, such as 'see what they do' or 'do the same as they did'. But rarely is there an explanation of exactly what you are supposed to be looking for, and what you are supposed to do with it once you find it. Another issue is, how are you to decide which dissertations will be the best models for you and your research topic?

However it is phrased, what the person (usually a supervisor or fellow student) is really advising you to do is this: closely analyze the organization, writing style, and formatting of successful dissertations, and use them as models for your own. I am a great believer in learning to write through close textual analysis of model pieces of writing (others and your own). So my purpose is to provide you with a set of dissertation models, show you what to look for, and help you to use what you learn strategically to write your own thesis. Woven throughout the chapters on writing up the thesis are examples from a set of six model dissertations that lead you through the structure, argument and writing/language conventions of the sections of a thesis. I have drawn on doctoral level work rather than Masters: a Masters thesis is similar in structure and content – the differences lie mainly in scale – and so I felt Masters students can benefit from doctoral models but that the reverse would not be true. I also felt that exposure to doctoral writing can provide Masters students with something of a roadmap towards completing a future project at the next academic level.

The dissertations were chosen to offer a range of topics and designs. Three are from the UK and three from Canada. To suggest the complex variety of advanced degrees that are currently available, I have included different types of doctorates: four traditional research doctorates; one professional practice doctorate; and one doctorate on the basis of published work. Here is a summary of the 'code' I use to refer to each author, her or his general topic, the research design and, in brackets, the type of doctorate:

> [KE] Karen Eisler: leadership practices of nurse managers, staff retention and quality of care; descriptive correlational [traditional doctorate]

> [JL] Jennifer Lynne Lapum: patient experiences of technology in open-heart surgery; narrative inquiry [traditional doctorate]

> [SJM] Sarah Jane McGeorge: older adults and mental health; constructivist grounded theory [doctorate in professional studies]

> [SM] Stephen Moore: anti-social behaviour in three social contexts; social constructivism [PhD on the basis of published work]

> [MRV] Munikumar Ramasamy Venkatasalu: cultural issues in health care; constructive grounded theory [traditional doctorate]

> [FWM] C. Faith Wight Moffatt: hypertensive pregnant women; RCT [traditional doctorate]

SOURCES

Eisler, K. (2009) 'The leadership practices of nurse managers and the association with nursing staff retention and the promotion of quality care in two Saskatchewan hospitals'. University of Toronto: Lawrence S. Bloomberg Faculty of Nursing.

Lapum, J.L. (2009) 'Patients' narratives of open-heart surgery: Emplotting the technological'. University of Toronto: Lawrence S. Bloomberg Faculty of Nursing.

McGeorge, S.J. (2011) 'Dynamic complexity: Invisible nursing: The construction of age-related complexity by registered nurses working in mental health services'. Teesside University: Doctorate in Professional Studies.

Moore, S. (2012) 'An exploration of the social construction of anti-social behaviour in the contexts of community, public transport and travel to school'. Anglia Ruskin University: Doctorate on the Basis of Published Work, Faculty of Health, Social Care and Education.

Venkatasalu, M.R. (2011) 'Understanding home, homeland, and family at the end of life: A qualitative study of older South Asians in East London'. University of Nottingham: Ph.D., School of Nursing, Midwifery, and Physiotherapy.

Wight Moffatt, C.F. (2009) 'A randomized controlled trial of the effects of guided imagery on blood pressure in hypertensive pregnant women'. University of Toronto: Ph.D., Lawrence S. Bloomberg Faculty of Nursing.

WHAT IS THE ROLE OF WRITING IN POST-GRADUATE STUDIES?

At the post-graduate level, students in Nursing and allied health professions engage in a variety of advanced writing forms that include papers on specialized topics for post-graduate courses, systematic literature reviews, grant proposals, conference presentations, publications, dissertations that report on research, and development of evidence-based practice. Through writing, these students demonstrate two dimensions of knowledge: 1) comprehensive knowledge of their field; and 2) the ability to expand the knowledge base of their profession through research, publication and leadership in practice.

- Reading, thinking and writing together form a single activity. Post-graduate programmes give you the time and space to develop all three.
- You become a member of a discourse community by learning to speak and use its language.
- You are changed by language and in turn your use of language will change the field as you create new knowledge.
- All writing is persuasive, and good writers wield power within society.
- Successfully writing a thesis is a watershed mark in your development, and it is a highly empowering experience.
- The discipline of reading/thinking/writing creates neural pathways that give you a precise eye for detail, the ability to hold larger amounts of information in your head, and the ability to analyze situations rapidly and effectively. This is indispensible for leadership roles in healthcare.

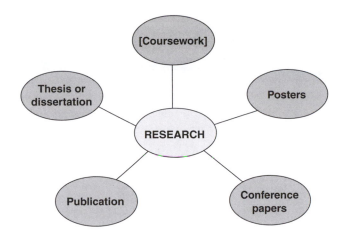

Figure 1.1   The wheel of post-graduate life

The following frameworks can help you understand the nature of a thesis-based degree in which you conduct research:

> *The Wheel:* Think of your post-graduate research interests as the hub of a wheel. The spokes of the wheel are all the things that both emerge from and contribute to your research: reading the literature, completing coursework (if relevant), writing your thesis; presenting at conferences and networking; preparing poster and paper presentations; publishing.
>
> *From Journeyman to Master:* The modern university has its roots in the mediaeval university, which was structured much like any other mediaeval guild. The three academic levels of undergraduate, post-graduate and professor/lecturer correspond to the guild ranks of apprentice, journeyman and master. In the modern university, undergraduate education seeks to provide a solid foundation of content and critical skills, along with the clinical skills required for registration to practise. At the Masters level, the focus is on acquiring a comprehensive knowledge of a field of practice knowledge, theory and research. The move from Masters to PhD level represents a major shift, from learning the field comprehensively at the Masters level to contributing something original to the field at the PhD level. The culmination of the process – the final initiation into the guild – is the doctoral thesis, which is accepted following a *viva voce* examination or defense. Your entry into the guild gives you the authority to take part in the discourse of the community. A way to think about discourse is as the 'community's dialogue about what it believes it knows and has a good basis for knowing' (Petre and Rugg, 2011, p.3). Discourse also refers to the ways in which the community engages in that dialogue, its unique vocabulary and ways of using language.

FOR FURTHER READING

Petre, M. and Rugg, G. (2011) *The Unwritten Rules of PhD Research* (2nd edn).
Maidenhead: McGraw-Hill/Open UP Study Skills.

WHAT DEGREE DO YOU WANT?

By this, I do not mean what letters would you like to see after your name. I mean that you need to match your aspirations and your strengths with your goals. Do you want a degree that prepares you for an academic research and teaching career? Organizational leadership? Leadership in clinical practice? Whatever your aspirations, it is important to analyze the different degree streams and decide what one will get you there. You also want to know what competencies you will be developing through the degree work and how well they match with your aptitudes. For example, you may feel a passion for improving the administrative frameworks under which hospital nurses conduct their practice, but if you are not well suited to the minutiae of managing projects and budgets, you will never achieve your goal. In the next section, we'll talk about things that help or block you from getting through to a successful conclusion.

An indispensable resource for anyone considering a post-registration degree in Nursing is the National Health Service's model of careers in Nursing, found on its website at http://nursingcareers.nhsemployers.org/. The site offers a Nursing Career Framework, an interactive tool in the form of a wheel that allows you to click on a particular pathway (mental health and psychosocial care; supporting long-term care; first contact, access and urgent care; acute and critical care; and family and public health), a type of degree within each pathway (research, education, management, and clinical), and finally career streams you can pursue with the degree. Clicking on any section of the wheel takes you to information about different types of jobs, the skills and competencies they involve, case studies from nurses working in these roles, and links to other resources. This framework is tremendously helpful, whether you are in the UK or not, because it is easily generalizable to the US, Canadian or Australian context. There is not a national framework for the US, where the post-registration degree landscape is highly complex and variable. In Canada, the Canadian Nurses Association offers a national framework for advanced nursing practice, and it describes competencies for advanced practice in clinical, research, leadership, and consultation and collaboration. It does not, however, offer the level of practical detail of the NHS framework.

An excellent source of information for American students contemplating a graduate degree is the American Association of Colleges of Nursing (AACN), a national organization of nurses that is dedicated exclusively to advancing nursing education. The association's brochure, *Your Guide to Graduate Nursing Programs*, will help you navigate the over 2000 graduate degree programmes offered in some 500 schools of nursing nationwide and understand your options for nursing education. Find it at www.aacn.nche.edu/publications/brochures/GradStudentsBrochure.pdf. It is especially valuable for making a decision between the traditional research-based PhD and the increasingly popular DNP (doctor of nursing practice), which prepares students for advanced clinical practice.

Nurses and allied health professionals hope for many things from a graduate degree, including: i) training for an academic teaching and/or research career; ii) training for research in professional settings; iii) high level training for a professional context; iv) a sense of intellectual curiosity and a desire for further education; and there are other reasons as well. Before you begin a degree programme, you need a clear picture of what you are entering into and why. Let's survey the landscape:

Masters-level programmes

Masters-level degrees in the health professions are frequently sought by individuals who have been in practice for some time since receiving their undergraduate education and professional accreditation. These degrees are sought because they have the potential to enhance individual career development, in a wide array of clinical practice, research, education and management settings.

A crucial difference in Nursing and health degrees in Canada and the US versus the UK and Australia lies in 'taught' (i.e., course-based) elements and the thesis element. At the Bachelor's (pre-registration) level in the UK/Australia, it is widely expected that students will write a lengthy (10,000–12,000 word) dissertation in their final year. In North America such a requirement is far from common. This distinction between taught and thesis extends to the Masters level as well (and to the doctoral level, as we'll see below). In North America, MSc programs that are entirely course-based are the norm, while in the UK and Australia, even taught degrees are likely to culminate in a thesis.

A taught programme is probably the most similar to an undergraduate degree in that the student takes a series of 'taught' courses, some required and some elective, and is assessed on them. For this reason, the taught Masters is not addressed in this book. There is a great deal of excellent advice on writing for courses in *Writing for Nursing and Midwifery Students* (Taylor, 2013). Typically, core required courses will focus on providing a grounding in research methods and evidence-based practice, while elective courses provide opportunities to explore fields of particular interest, such as population health, leadership, management, policy and many others. A taught programme may also contain a research or practical project, a thesis, or a placement. Where there is a thesis, a range of approaches is possible, including primary research, comprehensive literature reviews, and systemic or organizational reviews.

Some MSc programmes are research-based rather than taught. Although there may be some course requirements in research design, especially in North America, the purpose of a research degree is to conduct original research. Students may be required to undertake formal training in research at the start of the programme, but the precise focus and scope of the research are agreed upon between the student and a supervisor who will guide the student through the entire process of generating a research topic, questions and design, through the process of conducting the project and writing it up, and finally through to submission and defense. Generally, people take these programmes as a stepping stone to pursuing a research degree at the PhD level, and it is often possible to seamlessly 'convert' from a Masters to a PhD programme.

Doctoral-level programmes

Historically, the PhD in Nursing attracted only a small proportion of the profession and functioned to produce university professors and researchers. This has changed with the realization that a global shortage of nurses is already occurring and is widely predicted to grow with the aging of the population and the accompanying need for nursing care. The International Network for Doctoral Education in Nursing (INDEN), a non-profit professional association whose mission is to advance quality doctoral nursing education globally, lists doctoral nursing programmes in 32 countries; they include 20 in Australia, 13 in Canada (there are 15 as of 2010), 34 in the UK, and 133 in the US (Baker, 2010). INDEN identifies a large variety of doctoral education programmes, with the PhD being the most common. Traditionally, PhDs are research-based, but there is also a stream of doctoral education that is practice-based. The AACN (American Association of Colleges of Nursing) identifies two streams of doctoral education in the US: the DNP, which prepares nurses 'at the highest level of practice', and the PhD/DNS/DNSc, which prepare nurse researchers and academics. There are also a few hybrid doctoral programmes that combine a specialized professional practice component with a clinical dissertation. Similarly, in Australia, a Professional (Practice) Doctorate is available which combines coursework (about 33 per cent) and research (about 66 per cent). The research must make a significant contribution to knowledge and practice.

Very broadly speaking, on a global level there are two models of doctoral education in Nursing: UK/Australian and North American. Their broad pedagogical goals are the same: to produce the next generation of leaders in Nursing research, practice and management. They are rooted in shared theoretical frameworks, especially around ontology and epistemology. Both require the student to meet administrative deadlines; in other words, the responsibility for ensuring that all requirements of the programme are fulfilled in sequence lies with the student. Both models also ensure that someone within the faculty is responsible for guiding and monitoring the student's progress through the programme. Lastly, both models have some balance of coursework and research activities, but it is here that the differences begin to emerge.

In the UK and Australia, the system is based on personal tutor relationships, and the doctoral programme consists of a research project and a written dissertation, which is then judged by a panel of examiners in a viva (much more about the viva in Chapter 12). Course requirements are minimal, though some UK research funding councils may require them.

In the US and Canada, the PhD student begins with a set of required courses that includes at least one course in research methods. Coursework may occupy one or two years, during which time the student also produces a proposal for the doctoral research project. The mix of courses is designed to ensure comprehensive knowledge of the profession and a solid grounding in research design. At the end of the coursework period, the student must pass the 'comprehensives', oral and/or written examinations, which test the student's comprehensive knowledge base in the field. Once the comprehensives are passed and the proposal has been accepted, the research phase of the programme begins and the PhD 'student' becomes a PhD 'candidate'. In the final phase, the candidate undertakes a scholarly research project, which is then written up as a dissertation and defended before a committee (in many cases, especially in the US, the defense is open to anyone who wishes to attend). (Properly speaking, a 'thesis' is written at the Masters level and a 'dissertation' for a doctorate, but it is very common to use the word 'thesis' for both, as I do in this book.) The traditional thesis follows a single sustained narrative that moves from identifying a problem and research questions, discussing the research and theoretical literature, describing the research methodology, presenting results and discussing them. However, a new model is increasingly an option. In a 'publication thesis', introductory and discussion chapters frame a series of articles on the research that the candidate has successfully published. Within the stream of so-called 'professional' doctorates (i.e., doctorates that focus directly on addressing particular clinical, organizational or systemic issues), a thesis may develop and test an intervention rather than conduct a research study.

In the UK, there is traditionally a single supervisor. A co-supervision model is increasingly common, but one person will still be the primary supervisor. In North America, a supervisor and a committee oversee the research and thesis. In one common North American model, an Advisory Committee consists of one member of the graduate faculty as primary supervisor, who meets multiple times a year with the student, plus two or three other graduate faculty with related research interests. The full committee meets at least once a year in order to monitor the student's progress and document it in a written report. This is intended to provide positive direction for the research and ensure that issues are caught early and addressed, as well as to document the student's progress. In Australia, the student has a panel of supervisors, usually in a more distant relationship than a North American committee.

Whatever the supervisory structure is, make sure as part of your research into post-graduate programmes that the university or department has clear guidelines that lay out the responsibilities of supervisors and students to each other.

Undertaking a doctoral programme involves a considerable time commitment, anywhere from three to seven years. In the UK and Australia, national policies ensure that institutions encourage earlier times to completion (McAlpine and Amundsen, 2011, p.7). Certainly the expense involved and the overall inadequacy of funding sources such as scholarships or grants are also an encouragement to students to complete as quickly as possible.

FOR FURTHER READING

Baker, C. (2010) Doctoral Education in Nursing: Overview of doctoral education in nursing in an international context [PowerPoint].

CASN (2010) Doctoral Forum: Advancing the Canadian Vision. Canadian Association of Schools of Nursing. Available at: www.casn.ca/en/Past_Conferences_124/items/6.html

Green, H. (2005) 'Doctoral education in the UK: Trends and challenges'. Review paper prepared for Forces and Forms of Change in Doctoral Education International Conference, CIRGE, University of Washington, Sept.

Green, R. and Macauley, P. (2007) 'Doctoral students' engagement with information: An American-Australian perspective', *Libraries and the Academy* 7(3): 317–32.

McAlpine, L. and Amundsen, C. (2011) 'To be or not to be? The challenges of learning academic work', in L. McAlpine and C. Amundsen (eds) *Doctoral Education: Research-based strategies for doctoral students, supervisors and administrators* (pp.1–13). Springer Sciences+Business Media. doi 10.1007/978-94-007-0504-4.

WHY SOME SUCCEED AND OTHERS DO NOT

What do you bring with you when you enter a post-graduate programme, whether at the Masters or the doctoral level? In the uncertainty and anxiety of starting a new endeavour, it is easy to focus on your own deficits. I will speak here from long experience of one-on-one writing instruction with Nursing students at the beginning of their programme and say that the number one concern they express is worry about coming back to university and having to write. So if this is you, you are in good and plentiful company.

In fact, you bring with you many strengths that will be invaluable and greatly increase your chances of success. Green and Macauley (2007) speak here of students entering doctoral programmes in education, yet what they say is entirely applicable to Masters and doctoral students in the health professions as well:

> [They are] motivated by an imperative to improve their field's professional practice. As practitioners, they bring a high degree of experiential maturity, professional expertise, and accumulated wisdom to their study environment. Generally profiled as mature-age, accomplished professionals, they are fully aware of academic, workplace, and personal obligations; as such, they are skilled in negotiating multiple commitments and blending them when necessary. During the time of … study, the impetus to situate their identities simultaneously in communities of … education, professional practice, and their personal lives is quite compelling. (p.322)

Further, post-graduate students are cognitively mature and tend to be accomplished learners. That is, they understand their own learning styles and personal contexts, and readily develop appropriate strategies for learning in their new context.

Sadly, however, not everyone who enters post-graduate studies completes. Sometimes this is because of issues encountered during the programme, and we'll talk about those at the appropriate time, but it can also result from coming into post-graduate studies with faulty assumptions such as these:

Be practical: know what having a Masters or PhD can do for you in the real world

On a practical level, earning a Masters or PhD suggests to the world that it is safe to hire you to fill a university post or senior clinical or administrative position. As well, because global standards for receiving post-graduate degrees have many commonalities in rigour and requirements, they are highly portable. You can also expect, over the course of your career, to receive more money if you have one, but you cannot expect to walk into a high-paying job immediately after graduation. Note that I said 'over the course of your career'. As in any field, you will need to build a career.

This is especially true in the academic world. On-the-job, post-degree training is often required. For lecturer and professoriate positions, it is much cheaper for a university to hire faculty on limited-term contracts than on a tenured basis. Contracts also increase a department's control over academic offerings when faculty can be replaced with relative ease. But the rewards of an academic career, once established, are very gratifying – intellectual freedom; a great deal of scheduling freedom; good to excellent salary, benefits, and working conditions; and the satisfaction of doing good in the world by creating new knowledge and disseminating it to new generations of nurses and nurse researchers.

Don't come in with unrealistic expectations and then refuse to change them

Of course, the problem is that they don't seem at all unrealistic to you. Perhaps you have observed that there are too many medication errors in hospitals and you have great ideas for ending them once and for all. But then your supervisor rejects all your proposals to develop your ideas and put them into action, then wants you to do a statistical analysis of 15 years of data on medication errors in regional nursing homes. The two of you are in constant conflict and, in the end, you are the one to leave.

Don't think you will be revolutionizing healthcare

People are less likely to think this will happen as the result of their getting a Masters degree, but at the PhD level, one cause of great stress is a misunderstanding of the doctoral requirement for 'original work that makes a significant contribution'. It does not mean you are expected to change the world. Far from it. People who enter PhD studies with goals that are too lofty often sink under the weight of their own unrealistic expectations. My own graduate supervisor put it this way – doing a PhD means learning more and more about less and less. It is intuitive to imagine that the most important part of PhD research is the result. But one could argue that an even more important part of the process is demonstrating that you have learned how to ask questions about healthcare problems and how to go about answering them.

PhD research moves the discourse along; it does not need to revolutionize it. A good standard is to expect that PhD research should produce at least one paper in a peer-reviewed journal. In other words, your research should introduce you to the larger research community and enable you to engage with it as a full member. Think of it this way – your research will not revolutionize healthcare, but it is an important step in a career that very well might.

Don't fantasize about the scholarly life

It is certainly true that in a Masters or PhD programme you will experience great enjoyment in discussing complex ideas and issues with like-minded, smart, articulate colleagues, often over coffee or something stronger. But that happens only some of the time. Much of the time you will feel you are too busy to breathe. Sometimes you will hate your research, hate writing, and generally hate the world. Sometimes you will not go somewhere fun because you have to write, only to get almost nothing done. You will reach a point when, if one more person asks you when you'll be finished with all this because it does seem to be taking you forever, you may not be responsible for your actions. So if the main thing that comes to mind when you consider doing a post-graduate degree is some sort of fantasy about the intellectual life, you risk being overwhelmed by the day-to-day realities.

Don't confuse academic research with Wikipedia

One of the blessings of the internet is the vast amount of information it makes available to everyone. Another blessing is the sheer fun of internet research. Its fatal curse, though, from an academic point of view, is the lack of filters to separate reliable, valid information from the unreliable or simply false. Be prepared to devote a great deal of time to immersing yourself in academic publications, on as close to a daily basis as possible, in order to seek out and learn the strongest evidence-based knowledge.

Once you are in post-graduate studies, here are some attitudes and actions that will greatly improve your chances of successful completion:

> **Read. Read some more. Then read some more.** Read until you know which journals, which organizations (such as the WHO or NHS) and which authors/research teams are the most relevant and most interesting. Make sure you keep up with them on a regular basis – they form the foundation of the knowledge base you are building. Read widely around that core, exploring other journals, new authors. Find them through the reference lists in your core readings. Ask your supervisor and fellow students for new things to read.

Write. Write some more. Then write some more. The old piece of advice to write every day is still the best advice. Is it humanly possible to do that? Of course not (unless, of course, a deadline looms. Deadlines make heroes of us all). But remember that 'writing' casts a very broad net. If you are reading an article and you make some marginal notes, you have written that day. If you get an idea while you are in transit to work and you write it down so you don't forget it, you have written that day.

Be methodical on a day-to-day basis. Some examples: i) Build an annotated bibliography by making an entry every time you read something new. This is one of your most powerful research tools, and there is more about them in Chapter 3; ii) back up your work to an external drive (such as a memory stick) as your last action of the day. Do not tempt the fates by trusting that your computer will never, ever fail or be stolen; iii) maintain files of administrative papers in, for example, an accordion file or filing cabinet. Do not rely on the archaeological method of filing, also known as the pile on the floor.

Communicate with others. By 'others' I mean: i) your supervisor. Much more on that in Chapter 2; ii) a network, even a small one, of fellow students who can give you friendship and news; iii) an informal committee of specialists whose expertise you can draw on (such as librarians and statisticians), and others who are not necessarily specialists, but are intelligent people who are willing to read and discuss your work with you; iv) the larger research community through presenting at conferences and research days.

Don't hide in your office. Psychologically, it is very easy for writers to retreat into their own little world, isolated with their writing and all the problems it creates. This often combines with a fear of showing their writing to anyone else until it is 'ready', by which is meant 'perfect'. This can lead students to choose supervisors they are confident will not want to see frequent drafts, or to avoid submitting a draft until their supervisor must hound them for it. Hiding in your office also means not interacting with your colleagues in the programme – the very people who are going through exactly the same trials you are and who can be an excellent source of much-needed support and information.

STARTING THE RIGHT WAY

First, ensure that your **physical supports** are in place. Optimally, you should have a dedicated office space, preferably a room of its own. In choosing the space, consider whether you need quiet to work or whether you are one of those who can easily block out distractions. You should ensure you have shelf space for books, plus a filing cabinet for course papers and journal articles. The archaeological system of filing – that is, piles on the desk and floor that are added to as new materials come in – is a terrible time-waster and stressor when something must be found.

Then there are your **social supports**. Make sure you have a discussion with the significant others in your life, especially if you live with them. You will need their understanding when you have to cancel social occasions, as well as their assistance to take up day-to-day responsibilities you won't have time for. The time for these negotiations is before you start your studies, not in the middle when you – and they – are stressed by your workload. It is unwise to test your relationship by assuming they will be understanding and helpful in a situation with which they too are unfamiliar.

Finally, take advantage of your **institutional supports.** Does your institution have a writing centre or academic success centre that you are eligible to use? If so, make sure you use it. Professional writers, including your professors when they publish, regularly ask each other to be their readers. Why shouldn't you also benefit from having a trained eye look over what you've written? If that type of institutional support isn't available to you, draw on your fellow students, and reciprocate – our eye for our own work is sharpened by critiquing that of others. Draw also on your significant others as readers, and don't forget to reward their kindness with a kind word or deed of your own. Reading and commenting on an academic paper is not everyone's idea of a fun evening.

As soon as you receive your schedule, give serious consideration to how you will **manage your time**. Remember that the schedule you are given does not include the time you will need for reading, writing, study, travel, or simply the rest of your life. Don't assume, because you may in general be a good time manager, that everything will somehow get done on time. The work you are undertaking is new. It is easy to underestimate the amount of time you will need to keep up with all the reading. This is especially true during your first term in a programme.

Choosing times to schedule for study and writing needs some thought. Base your decisions not only on what times are available to you but also on what times are most efficient for you. Are you sharpest in the morning, or are you a night owl? Are you able to read while in transit?

A strategy that many find helpful is to map out a large calendar sheet for the term and hang it in your work space. Colours are helpful to indicate different types of work. Don't forget to include social occasions and small rewards for your hard work, such as a nice dinner out at mid-term or a weekend away at the end of term. The calendar is intended to reduce your stress, not add to it, so if you find you are not able to follow the schedule you set, be flexible about making changes to reflect the reality you are experiencing.

DEVELOPING THE SUPERVISORY RELATIONSHIP AND OPPORTUNITIES FOR FUNDING

OVERVIEW

- What and who is a supervisor?
- Choosing a supervisor
- What to discuss during your initial meetings
- The time to ask questions is now ...
- Working with your supervisor: a mid-programme reality check
  - Questions to ask yourself
  - What to do if problems arise ...
- Money never hurts: ten tips for funding applications

The health professions need university graduates who are not only technically skilled, but also able to conceptualize social and ethical issues, shape policy, fulfil advocacy roles, and communicate their expertise to a wide range of healthcare stakeholders. As a student, you can expect to gain knowledge, as well as to become a member of a knowledge community.

Although this is a book about writing, as its title promises, it is just as much a book about the experience of being a post-graduate student, because that is the context in which your writing will take place. (Think of it as a timeline and survival manual.) The post-graduate student experience is transformative, especially at the doctoral level. You are making an enormous personal investment and will never be the same person again.

In many ways, post-graduate studies are like a board game. You make your way around a winding path where you can't see around the turns. For some periods of time, you move along smoothly, then enter a period when your way is blocked. Sometimes you land on a reward; sometimes on a loss or setback. The reward or setback may result from a decision you made or may simply be luck, good or ill. Sometimes you miscalculate in your strategy, perhaps because of factors you couldn't know about; other times your strategy succeeds. There is even a set of winners and of losers. There are those for whom the post-graduate degree results in everything they'd hoped for. Some people the degree sends in a new but ultimately better direction. And, sad to say, some don't complete the game or experience no good result, despite all the effort put in.

But given the fact that inadequate supervision is widely cited as a major reason why students fail to complete doctoral programmes (the issue seems not to have been studied at the Masters level), it is time to take a close look at that relationship – how to plant the seeds of a good one and how to nurture it to fruition.

WHAT AND WHO IS A SUPERVISOR?

In an academic context, what exactly does a supervisor do?

A supervisor has two major, equally important responsibilities. A supervisor is a researcher, and your ability to produce research is important to her or his career. A supervisor is a graduate faculty member who has primary responsibility for helping you learn the art and science of research, as well as for guiding you successfully through to completion of your degree (*SGS Guidelines*, 2012). As the University of Toronto School of Graduate Study guidelines describe it, good post-graduate supervision can be recognized by a number of characteristics:

> It should inspire and guide students to reach their full scholarly potential. It should provide an environment that is supportive yet stimulating. It should enable students to learn the essential methodologies, concepts, and culture of their discipline, and perform research of high quality and significance. It should introduce them to the wider context of the discipline and the relevant communities of scholars, and help position them for future careers both within and outside academe. It should foster a strong sense of academic integrity. And it should help students successfully navigate the journey through their program with a clear understanding of the appropriate requirements, rules and procedures, and with any emerging problems handled in a timely fashion with compassion and clarity. (p.3)

There is an important third element: in a good working relationship, in which both sides are open and tolerant of each other, the supervisor is also your teacher, responsible for training you to conduct advanced research and write about it. As we'll see below, the teaching extends to training you take on a role within the 'discourse community' of researchers. The balance of the two roles depends on whether the supervisor sees her or himself primarily as a researcher or as a teacher. There is another important element of your relationship together, which supervisors fulfil with varying degrees of skill – acting as a mentor, taking an interest in you as a person and giving you the benefit of their own experiences 'in the trenches' of the professional and academic worlds. The supervisor should direct students to resources so they can gain comprehensive knowledge, and advise them on the administrative process. The quality of the work that a student produces reflects on the supervisor as well, so the relationship is a career-related one on both sides.

There is a wide spectrum of supervisory styles. Some maintain close contact with their students, perhaps meeting weekly with the whole group of the supervisor's post-graduate students and individually on a frequent basis. Such a mentoring supervisor will support and enrich their students' experience, and introduce them to people in their academic community, in person whenever possible or at least through their work. In other words, they see it as their duty to provide as much emotional support and academic guidance as possible. On the far other end, some see their students as, essentially, independent researchers and provide only occasional feedback and direction.

The supervisory relationship is one of the most important but under-discussed aspects of the post-graduate student experience. That one relationship can make or break the experience you have as a post-graduate student. That is not to say that it is the only relationship of importance to students – in research on doctoral education, students emphasize the role of a range of individuals beyond the supervisor (McAlpine and Amundsen, 2011, p.3) – but it is clearly a crucial one. For some, their supervisor becomes a lifelong friend and mentor. For others, their supervisor seems like a punishment sent by some vengeful fate. For most, of course, the relationship falls somewhere between those extremes.

The negative consequences of a failure to complete are much greater for students than their supervisors, which means that it is up to you to ensure you get the supervision you need and are entitled to.

CHOOSING A SUPERVISOR

Policies vary widely among post-graduate programmes in regard to the formal arrangement between a supervisor and her or his students. In some cases, especially at the Masters level, the supervisor is, quite simply, assigned by the department. These decisions are generally made at meetings of the department's admissions committee, where individual professors will express their preference for the students they would like to take on, or are available to take on. In other programmes, students arrange meetings with professors they feel might be the most appropriate supervisor for their research interests, and come to an agreement with one of them. This is not always as free a choice as one might hope – in small departments, there may be only one professor researcher in the area of the student's interest. Sometimes the choosing of a supervisor comes after the student has been in the programme doing coursework for some months; in other cases, they need a professor's agreement to be their supervisor as part of the admissions requirements. Whatever the mechanism, once the supervisor–student relationship is formally set, it is difficult to change supervisors. For this reason, it is important for you to be as actively engaged in the process as your institution allows and to be clear – both in your own mind and in your statements to a potential supervisor – about what you hope to gain from the relationship and what you can contribute to it.

It could be argued that the most advantageous position from which to be seeking a supervisor is one in which you've been in your programme for a while doing coursework. This gives you the opportunity to get to know the relevant faculty and their reputations, and to speak to their current post-graduate students.

Here are some tips for choosing a supervisor:

1. On the department's website, check their online bios, CVs, publications, organizational affiliations, research grants held, honours and awards they've received. If they are part of a research group, see what the aims and activities of the group have been.

2. Don't forget to check blogs, discussion groups, or social media sites that they may contribute to, in order to have a more personal perspective than the formal documentation of a CV can offer.

3. Read their publications to decide if their research interests align with your own.

4. Using an online citation index, track the number of times they are cited by other scholars, which will give you a sense of their relative impact within the research and academic community.

5. Contact the departmental administrator for the email addresses of the supervisor's current and recent students. Email and ask to meet (and buy them a drink or a light meal). Ask them their perceptions of the supervisor's 'style', how it is working with them, and if there have been problems, such as students who completed but with difficulty and a lot of interpersonal conflict. Meeting with the current students will also give you a sense of whom you may turn to throughout your programme for advice, feedback and support. You can ask recent graduates how much help the supervisor gave them in finding a job and/or building a professional network.

6. Make an appointment to speak to the department administrator or post-graduate programme coordinator. These people can inform you about the faculty members who are your potential supervisors. They may also be able to tell you how many of her/his students fail to complete, or need to apply for extensions, and how this compares with other supervisors. They also have intimate knowledge of the programme requirements and policies. While it is true that your supervisor is available to advise you on these matters, it is also important to establish an early working relationship with the actual administrators.

7. Most important, perhaps, is meeting face-to-face with potential supervisors. When you do, pay attention to your instincts. Is this someone you feel you can like and trust? Someone you look forward to working with and learning from? Someone who seems to 'get' you?

WHAT TO DISCUSS DURING YOUR INITIAL MEETINGS

Make sure you take notes! Review them soon after a meeting and get back to the supervisor with questions or requests for clarification. Write down those answers too.

- Your thesis topic: you may or may not finalize your topic during these meetings, but you should feel comfortable with your range of choices. Thesis topics should be a good fit with the supervisor's larger research expertise; they should also reflect your genuine interest in particular topics.
- Ways of researching your topic: what research design[s] is your supervisor recommending? Is this a way of approaching the topic that appeals to you?

- Funding: where is your funding going to come from? The supervisor's research grant? Grants that you will apply for from government or other sources?
- Will you have teaching responsibilities? (This is a widespread expectation in North American universities.) If so, what will they be and how much time will you be devoting to them?
- Courses: if there is a coursework component, discuss the courses you will be required to complete. Are there additional courses the supervisor recommends, and why?
- If there will be a supervisory committee, ask questions about it. In North America, the supervisory committee generally consists of the supervisor plus two to three other graduate faculty members. The committee's major role is to meet with the student at set intervals to assess her or his progress and report on it. They also approve the final thesis, and take part in the defense. Ask how and when your committee will be chosen, and who your supervisor would recommend sit on it. Ask how often you will be meeting with them. Find out if they will also, on an ongoing basis, provide advice and feedback that complements and adds to the supervisor's.

THE TIME TO ASK QUESTIONS IS NOW ...

... to a potential supervisor:

- How many of your students successfully complete without needing an extension beyond the normal length of the programme?
- How many students have you worked with? How many do you have now? How many do you typically supervise at a time? (Remember that there is no formal process for learning to be a supervisor – faculty learn it by adapting their own experience as post-graduate students and/or by speaking with their colleagues about their own best practices. So if the person is new to supervision, you might ask them about how they were supervised during their own training.)
- What clinical skills support will I receive while doing my degree?
- Do you have long-range plans for the next number of years that might impact our work together (e.g., a sabbatical leave or retirement)? If so, what arrangements would be made to ensure continuity in my supervision?
- [if relevant] When and how will my committee be chosen? How often should I expect to meet with them? What is their input during the research and writing process? Will any of them advise me during the research and writing process, or are you my only source for feedback?
- Questions about your 'style' of working with your students: How often will we meet? Who will arrange the meetings? Can we communicate informally between meetings (i.e., when I have questions)?
- As part of the supervisor's research 'culture,' will I be working independently on a project of my own, or in a group as part of a larger research project?
- Questions about on-campus office space: Where will I work and what equipment will I have?

- Will you advise me on opportunities to present my work at conferences and research days? Do you have any sources of travel funding for post-graduate students?
- Will I be publishing during the programme? If so, when and how much is expected? Will you advise me on how to write up my research for publication and where to submit it? Will you advise me on the publication process? What about authorship? Do you typically take senior authorship?

… to the department:

- What are the milestones I must achieve throughout the programme and when? How will I be evaluated at each milestone?
- What (if any) courses am I required to take?
- What kind of examinations will I have and when? What will they be testing and what form do they take?
- In North America, it is common practice for the supervisor to be supplemented by a committee of (usually) three other graduate faculty. If this is the case, when and how is the committee formed, how often will I be meeting with them, and what role will they play?
- Does the department play a role in financial support throughout my programme? Does the department offer any support if I do not complete before other funding ends?
- Are travel funds for conferences available? (If available, these may be minimal, but every bit helps when you are a post-graduate student!)

… to yourself:

- Have I entered all administrative deadlines in my personal calendar?
- Do I have a schedule set for meetings with my supervisor?
- Am I taking a thorough set of notes during our initial meetings? Do I review them within a day of the meeting and ask the supervisor for clarification where needed?
- Once we have finalized all the expectations of our relationship on both sides, do we have them in writing? This may be a formal document required or encouraged by the department, or it may simply be an email summary. But the only way to be sure in future of what was agreed between you is to have it in written form.
- And last, but not least, do I feel excited about working with this supervisor?

SOURCES

Chen, S. (2011) 'Making sense of the doctoral dissertation defense: A student-experience-based perspective', in L. McAlpine and C. Amundsen (eds) *Doctoral Education: Research-based strategies for doctoral students, supervisors and administrators* (pp.97–114). Dordrecht, The Netherlands: Springer.

(Continued)

(Continued)

Green, H. (2005) 'Doctoral education in the UK: Trends and challenges'. Review paper prepared for Forces and Forms of Change in Doctoral Education International Conference. CIRGE, University of Washington.

Green, R. and Macauley, P. (2007) 'Doctoral students' engagement with information: An American-Australian perspective', *Libraries and the Academy* 7(3): 317–32.

McAlpine, L. and Amundsen, C. (2011) 'To be or not to be? The challenges of learning academic work', in L. McAlpine and C. Amundsen (eds) *Doctoral Education: Research-based strategies for doctoral students, supervisors and administrators* (pp.1–13). Dordrecht, The Netherlands: Springer.

McAlpine, L. and Amundsen, C. (eds) (2011) *Doctoral Education: Research-based strategies for doctoral students, supervisors and administrators*. Dordrecht, The Netherlands: Springer.

Paré, A. (2011) 'Speaking of writing: Supervisory feedback and the dissertation', in L. McAlpine and C. Amundsen (eds) *Doctoral Education: Research-based strategies for doctoral students, supervisors and administrators* (pp.59–74). Dordrecht, The Netherlands: Springer.

Petre, M. and Rugg, G. (2011) *The Unwritten Rules of PhD Research* (2nd edn). Maidenhead: McGraw-Hill/Open UP Study Skills.

SGS Guidelines (2012) *Graduate Supervision: Guidelines for students, faculty, and administrators* (2nd edn). Toronto, Canada: School of Graduate Studies, University of Toronto. Available at www.sgs.utoronto.ca/governance/policies.htm

Starke-Myerring, D. (2011) 'The paradox of writing in doctoral education: Student experiences', in L. McAlpine and C. Amundsen (eds) *Doctoral Education: Research-based strategies for doctoral students, supervisors and administrators* (pp.75–95). Dordrecht, The Netherlands: Springer.

WORKING WITH YOUR SUPERVISOR: A MID-PROGRAMME REALITY CHECK

Questions to ask yourself

- Am I making sure I maintain regular contact with my supervisor? Or am I waiting for her/him to ask how I'm doing? Am I avoiding contact because I think I haven't got enough work done and s/he'll be upset?
- When I email, do I get upset if s/he doesn't answer the same day?
- Do I send a draft of each chapter or do I 'save up' a large section and send it at the end of the term? (This is not a good strategy – remember that supervisors generally have teaching responsibilities and their heaviest marking loads come at the end of a term.)
- Do I get in touch a couple of weeks before I intend to send a draft? Do I ask if that's good timing for her/him and what sort of turn-around time s/he anticipates?
- How much direction am I getting? Does my supervisor micromanage me and my research so that I feel stifled? Or is the opposite true – s/he

pays no attention to me and I feel at sea without a rudder? Or are we at a balance somewhere between that I'm comfortable with?

- What is the quality of written feedback I'm getting on my drafts? Vague comments such as 'good' or 'needs more' aren't terribly helpful. Metaphors such as 'can you punch this up a little?' or 'needs better flow' express some vague goal (being punched up; flowing) but not how to get there.
- When I receive written feedback that I feel is negative, do I set it aside for at least one day before looking at it objectively (as though it applied to another person) and deciding if I still feel it is negative? Do I wait at least one more day before I send an email to ask for clarification?
- How am I progressing in the aspects beyond the research and thesis, such as publication, conferences, networking, funding?
- How would I assess the power dynamic in our relationship? Is it a negative factor (uncaring expert putting novice down) or is it a positive one (stimulating expert helping novice to learn)?
- Am I receiving the quality and quantity of emotional support that I want and can reasonably expect?
- Have I been careful to deal with small issues as they arise? Have I approached my supervisor respectfully while being clear about my concerns?
- Just as I expect my supervisor to let me know of any extended absences or delays, have I been careful to reciprocate?
- Just as I expect my supervisor to respect that I am often busy and under great stress, have I been careful to reciprocate?
- Based on all of the above, am I generally happy (perhaps with exceptions I can live with) about my relationship with my supervisor and my progress through the programme?

What to do if problems arise ...

Here as elsewhere in life, it's obviously best to deal with issues early on, when a little flexibility and compromise are generally all that is needed. Often, apparent problems are simply the result of miscommunication and vanish with a request for clarification. Students are often uneasy about approaching their supervisor in this way. This is because, even in the most collegial of student/faculty relationships, there is still a power dynamic at work. Students from cultures with a tradition of deference to authority may find initiating these discussions especially difficult. But whether your background has taught you to defer to authority or to challenge it, a respectful and open approach will almost always produce results.

First, identify the problem clearly in your own mind. What exactly is troubling you?

S/he doesn't answer my emails

Not at all? Or just not very quickly? Exactly how long does s/he take? Have you considered that s/he has a workload that is at least as heavy as your own? If your question was particularly important, did you indicate that in your original email?

S/he takes way too long to return my drafts

What does 'way too long' mean? Did you ask for a turnaround time when you submitted? What are you doing while you wait? If you are working ahead on your next chapter, you have less time to worry about the wait. It is not reasonable to expect a response in less than a week; two or even three weeks is a more likely time period. But if your supervisor takes longer than three weeks, or consistently misses her or his estimates on turnaround without any explanation, it's time to speak up. Ask if the submission schedule the two of you had agreed upon needs to be changed.

S/he doesn't seem to like me. S/he's always impatient with me

As emotional beings, we are all different. Some of us prefer less personal connection than others, or have been trained to believe it is inappropriate within an academic relationship. Speak to the supervisor's other students. Perhaps this is what s/he is like with everyone. If that is not the case, ask yourself if you are perhaps misinterpreting her or his words and actions.

I don't understand any of her comments on my drafts

Does this happen every time? Do you really not understand 'any' of the comments? Identify them and exactly what you are not understanding about each one. If there are too many for you to ask about in an email, ask for a meeting to go through them.

S/he makes way too many corrections to my writing - I feel I don't have any freedom to write what I want

Some supervisors feel it is their responsibility to guide your development as a writer with as much feedback as possible; others feel it is your responsibility to present them with as 'perfect' a draft as possible. Either way, this is simply their style of supervision. If, though, you find it too difficult to absorb so many comments, you could ask the supervisor to identify patterns of errors rather than every individual error.

S/he makes hardly any comments on my drafts. I want to know the right way to do things and I need more direction than I'm getting

What type of comments is s/he making? Are they suggestions for methodology or requests that you add something to the research itself? Are they comments on the way you have structured the draft (e.g., something should be moved to another section)? Are they 'mechanical' corrections to do with grammar, punctuation, referencing, and/or style? Not all supervisors comment in all these areas. Once you identify the kinds of comments being made and consider what kinds of comments you would like to have, you can approach him or her to discuss what is most helpful to you.

Sometimes the comments contradict each other, either somewhere else in the draft or in a previous draft

Changes to a previous draft may change the direction of the supervisor's comments. If there are apparent contradictions within the same draft, however, try to understand why the two contexts may be different. If you still can't resolve the contradiction, send an email to ask for clarification.

S/he doesn't seem to understand how much stress I am under

A supervisor is not the same as a counsellor, and while many are comfortable with a mentoring, counselling role, many are not comfortable or do not feel it is appropriate. Indeed, if you need counselling for stress, the best approach is to take advantage of support services offered by your university.

S/he has suddenly introduced something new s/he wants me to do in the research. S/he never mentioned this before

Ask for an explanation. It may be that you have already made some changes in your research design that make a new approach desirable or necessary. Or maybe it's because some aspect of your current design is not working out and must be rethought. Whatever the reason for the change, if it had been needed sooner, s/he would have mentioned it sooner.

[for North American students] S/he and my committee are telling me to do opposite things. There is a lot of animosity between them and I feel stuck in the middle. Whatever I do is wrong with somebody!

Ultimately, the person who has to resolve this potentially toxic situation is your supervisor. If it absolutely cannot be resolved, it is time for you to speak to the graduate coordinator for the department. The approach to take is to emphasize the effect the situation is having on your ability to complete your research and therefore your programme. Do NOT launch into a complaint about personalities, but be prepared to emphasize that there are personality conflicts that cannot be resolved, without getting into any more detail than you are asked for.

The relationship has turned completely toxic. I feel s/he is deliberately holding me back, as if s/he doesn't care if I get my degree or not, OR we simply cannot agree on my research and no compromise is possible

This complete breakdown in the relationship is the worst-case scenario. If none of your best efforts to resolve the situation have worked, speak to various levels of the administration. Start with your committee members (if you have a committee) and move progressively up the levels to the post-graduate coordinator for the programme, to the post-graduate dean of the faculty and, if needed, to the central university administration responsible for post-graduate programmes. You will also need emotional support from friends and family. Speak to your fellow students about your situation, and consult with university support professionals who are trained to help students deal with crisis situations. Possibly a mechanism can be found for you to transfer to a different supervisor, although this is often difficult to accomplish. Other faculty members may understandably be cautious about entering into such an emotionally charged situation, or may feel that they lack the expertise on your research topic to guide you. I hope you never get to the point of needing this final piece of advice, but here it is: Do not give up and withdraw from the programme unless you are certain you have exhausted all avenues for resolution. You are the biggest loser when that happens.

MONEY NEVER HURTS: TEN TIPS FOR FUNDING APPLICATIONS

You will have noticed that the topic of funding came up more than once in this chapter. This is because, at least once during your programme, you will be applying for funding. It may be a small amount to let you register for a local conference or cover some of your travel expenses for one in another city. It may be a modestly substantial amount to help you conduct a research project. Or it may be a large amount to cover your tuition and living expenses for the entire year. The latter is commonly a necessity for North American students in doctoral programmes; even at the Masters level, scholarships and bursaries are typically available.

But whether you are applying for a few pounds or dollars, or for many thousands of them, the principles and pitfalls of applying for money are the same.

A great deal of advice is available on writing applications for funding, grants or scholarships, both in workshops offered by university research offices and individual departments, and in published form such as Holtzclaw et al.'s (2009) *Grant Writing Handbook for Nurses*. Check the resources available to you and make good use of them. Here, however, is a distillation of all that advice to get you started:

1. **Read the application form**. Do exactly what it says. Do not omit anything; do not add anything. And do it in the order asked for. Don't make the committee hunt around for what they need, because it wastes their time and is annoying.

2. **Learn about the organization you are applying to.** Pay attention to their grant objectives and criteria; make sure that you and your research, or programme of study, are a good fit. Tailor your application accordingly. Also make sure you say something about the organization in your cover letter – committees can smell a generic application (where an identical letter and materials are sent out to multiple organizations). It makes you seem lazy and uninterested in them except for their money.

3. **Be succinct. More is not better.** Do write to the maximum length allowed but fill it with substance, not fluff. Also, don't fall for the myth that long, jargon-filled sentences make you seem knowledgeable and professional. You are actually being turgid and hard to understand – you bore the committee and/or leave them confused.

4. **Why you?** Why should they give money to you? What is it in your background, personal history, training, work and/or volunteer experience that makes you the candidate they are looking for?

5. **Show, don't tell.** Don't trot out a string of cliches ('I am a passionate, dedicated, hard-working, well-organized individual.') Instead, demonstrate those qualities: 'I have organized a national conference for student midwives, and my hard work and dedication were rewarded with a permanent seat on the association's council.'

6. **Persuade them, don't just describe.** If you seek funding for a research project, the committee needs a clear description of the project but will also want to be persuaded that:

- your problem is worthy of study and you are well-positioned to study it
- you have clear, precise objectives that can reasonably be achieved with the resources available to you
- you have good reasons for choosing your particular methodology
- you can complete your project in a timely fashion within a reasonable budget
- your results will contribute meaningfully to practice, research and/or theory
- you have effective plans to disseminate the knowledge your project generates

7. **Be honest.** Have there been any interruptions, delays or other setbacks in your progress to date? Don't leave the committee wondering – it breeds suspicion that you are hiding something. In contrast, an honest explanation will not hurt you and can even work in your favour.

8. **Ask a colleague or supervisor for a critical review of your application.** Take advantage of all the expertise available to you.

9. **Present them with an attractive package.** Proofread, double proofread, and ask someone else to proofread. Many an application has sunk beneath the weight of errors in grammar, punctuation, formatting and spelling. Never rely on a computerized spell-checker (which will be perfectly happy if, for example, you keep spelling 'health' as 'heath'). Format the application to be easy to read, with a 12-pt font, 1-inch margins all round, and text that's broken up into paragraphs. A little white space makes reading easier – remember, the eyes of overworked committees get *very* tired from long hours of reading.

10. **Keep trying.** Success is sweet but failure is common. Don't be discouraged; above all, don't take the rejection personally. Pick yourself up and find someone else to apply to.

FOR FURTHER READING

Holtzclaw, B.J., Kenner, C. and Walden, M. (2009) *Grant Writing Handbook for Nurses* (2nd edn). Sudbury, MA: Jones and Bartlett.

3

CRITICAL READING AND WRITING: ESSENTIAL STRATEGIES

OVERVIEW

- Build your bibliography
- Annotated (critical) bibliography
- The active reading process for a journal article
  - Questions to ask about each article you are reading
  - Final suggestions
- Types of literature you will be reading
  - Scholarly literature
  - Grey literature
  - Primary vs. secondary literature
  - Professional literature
- Strategies for the writing process
- Procrastination, writer's block and other barriers

BUILD YOUR BIBLIOGRAPHY

In the last chapter, I said that reading is an activity you will continuously engage in through your entire programme, and I suggested asking your supervisor in your early meetings for a list of essential reading to get you started.

Initially, you read in order to learn what is known about your research area. Later, you will read to learn what is NOT known in order to set your own research questions. And then, if you are a doctoral student, you will read to keep up-to-date and to be sure no one has scooped your research project. (This is something doctoral students must always be on the watch for. It could make it necessary for you to change your entire topic, or at least your methodology, even if you are already far advanced in your own work.)

One estimate is that established researchers have a core repertoire of 100 to 150 works which they know well and draw on readily (Petre and Rugg, 2011, p.69). The particular number doesn't really matter. Nor will that core repertoire consist only of works directly related to your particular specialization. Your time in post-graduate studies gives you a space in which to accumulate the comprehensive knowledge base that will inform the rest of your career. It is a time to allow intellectual curiosity to draw you from one piece of writing to another, sometimes landing you far afield of where you started. When you start reading in the afternoon and suddenly realize the sun is setting, that is when you know you are engaged with the intellectual world. Enjoy it – you may never have this opportunity again.

Considering how much and how widely they are reading, many students ask how they will ever retain it all in such a way that they can easily draw on it. How is it that effective researchers are able to do this? The answer is to build an annotated bibliography, starting from the beginning of post-graduate studies. For one thing, it builds your ability to search for and locate the literature. (Strategies for searching the research literature are discussed in detail in Chapter 7.) Second, the deliberate act of writing that the bibliographic process entails is a highly effective memory device. A side benefit is that it also saves time by helping you avoid duplicate searches and starting to read the same material twice. When you locate an apparently new source, a simple check of your bibliography will confirm whether it is new or not. You may choose to re-read it, but you won't waste time in case you don't.

Finally, the bibliography is an organizational and memory tool. It is not the same as an in-depth analysis of the sources you choose for your literature review. But it will be an indispensable resource when the time comes to conduct that review.

SOURCE

Petre, M. and Rugg, G. (2011) *The Unwritten Rules of PhD Research* (2nd edn). Maidenhead: McGraw-Hill/Open UP Study Skills.

ANNOTATED (CRITICAL) BIBLIOGRAPHY

An annotated bibliography is a record of the books and articles you have read, with a brief summary and comment on the content and usefulness of each. As the number of entries builds, you can subdivide the bibliography by subject. Increasingly, university libraries offer free citation software to students, and there are numerous products available commercially. These often feature a bibliography function that allows you to easily maintain an ongoing record of sources you have consulted, along with your brief comment about this source, and what it might be useful for. Whether you build your bibliography using citation software or manually on your own computer, the bibliography will be an invaluable resource as your programme progresses and the volume of your readings goes up.

A bibliography (also called an annotated or critical bibliography) is a set of individual entries, as short as a reference citation plus a couple of sentences, or as long as a page or more. Entries follow a simple three-part structure: citation, summary, and comment.

Each entry is headed by a full citation (author, date, title, publisher) in proper APA or Harvard reference style. This is done to allow you to easily retrieve the work at a later time without doing another search. (There is also the possibility that you will not find it in a second search – this is a trick of the universe designed to drive tired researchers mad.) It also allows you to cut-and-paste (or, in the case of reference managing software, retrieve) the entry into the reference list of your thesis or any papers you write.

A brief summary of the contents follows. For example, in the case of a research study, a summary could include some or all of these:

- the purpose or question
- the study design
- the theoretical framework, if it is stated
- the methods
- the important result[s]
- what they concluded
- their limitations
- what next research steps they recommend

The bibliography entry ends with a comment on the 'usefulness' of the work. What, on this reading, is the most important idea or fact that you take from it? For what purpose would this work be most helpful to you?

Behind these three simple steps, however, lie important critical skills that the bibliographic process forces you to develop: reading, attention to detail, and analysis. This is especially true when sources are advancing ideas and arguments, as opposed to reporting on what was done and found during a research study.

Reading may seem an obvious skill. We were all taught to do it at a young age. But it is precisely this 'taken-for-granted' nature of reading that can prevent us from seeing that the rigorous, structured reading of a post-graduate programme is different from the reading we do for enjoyment or information. Not understanding this leads to frustration at the amount of time spent reading, relative to the result. An inability to read efficiently and effectively is sometimes a reason for leaving a post-graduate programme altogether, with a devastating sense of having 'failed' at a skill that apparently any child can conquer.

The best writers are adept at what is called 'close textual analysis', that is, the ability to pull apart the argument and language use of the texts they read. Broadly speaking, there are two types of close reading: **content** and **critical**. We read for content when we want to know how to assemble a piece of equipment, or what the statistics were on coronary disease in 2008. Content reading means reading for information. It employs what we call 'closed thinking'.

Critical reading means reading for idea and argument. We read critically when we want to make judgements about *how* a text is argued and what that argument is. It employs what we call 'open thinking'.

There is also a difference between **passive** reading and **active** reading. We read magazines or social media passively, sitting still as we absorb the content of one article or item and move on to the next. But when we read in order to write, the process becomes active. We physically engage with the material by writing on it and making notes about it. We integrate the activities of thinking and writing into the reading process.

THE ACTIVE READING PROCESS FOR A JOURNAL ARTICLE

If there is an abstract, read it first to gain a good summary understanding of the article.

Skim through the article, especially the introduction and conclusion, just to see the names of headings and get a sense of the article's structure. You'll also get a sense of which of the sections are most important.

Next, read the article right through once or twice passively, until you feel you have a good understanding of its contents. Never start copying sentences or passages that look useful without reading the article right through at least once. This is because writers will typically make the same point in a variety of positions, from different perspectives or in relation to different evidence. It is better to wait until you identify these different iterations of the point and can summarize or paraphrase them using words of your own, rather than just passively copying.

Now pick up a pen or highlighter. Go through the article carefully to underline, bracket or highlight key words, concepts, phrases or sentences. Engage with the material by making marginal notations or jotting down ideas/questions/points related to the topic. Pay particular attention to the first sentences of sections and paragraphs – it is in these 'topic sentences' that writers state directly what point is about to be made.

Read for understanding of their ideas and evidence, as well as to spark your own thoughts and questions about the article.

Questions to ask about each article you are reading

1. Who is the author or authors? What universities and/or research organizations are they affiliated with? Am I seeing any pattern in terms of where the high-quality research is being conducted and by whom?
2. Has the author formulated a problem/issue?
3. Is the problem/issue ambiguous or clearly articulated? Is its significance (scope, severity, relevance) discussed?
4. What are the strengths and limitations of the way the author has formulated the problem or issue?
5. Could the problem have been approached more effectively from another perspective?
6. What is the author's research orientation (e.g., interpretive, critical science, combination)?
7. What is the author's theoretical framework (e.g., psychoanalytic, developmental, feminist)?
8. What is the relationship between the theoretical and research perspectives?
9. Has the author evaluated the literature relevant to the problem/issue? Does the author include literature that takes positions s/he does not agree with?

10. In a scientific research study, how good are the three basic components of the study design (i.e., population, intervention, outcome)? How accurate and valid are the measurements? Is the analysis of the data accurate and relevant to the research question? Are the conclusions validly based upon the data and analysis?
11. In popular literature, does the author use appeals to emotion, one-sided examples, rhetorically charged language and tone? Is the author objective, or is s/he merely 'proving' what s/he already believes?
12. How does the author structure his or her argument? Can you 'deconstruct' the flow of the argument to analyze if/where it breaks down?
13. Is this a book or article that contributes to your understanding of the problem under study, and in what ways is it useful for theory or practice? What are its strengths and limitations?
14. How does this book or article fit into the topic or research question you are exploring?

Final suggestions

A bibliography is most useful if it is periodically reviewed, especially a day or two after you create the entry. Re-read the entry, pretending you've never read the original article, and ask yourself two questions: am I getting everything I need to know to understand the overall content of this article, and am I getting a sense of its overall quality and usefulness?

A related activity to building a bibliography is building a glossary of terms. This is a suggestion often made to non-native speakers of English in order to improve their vocabulary. However, it is equally useful to native speakers learning the technical and theoretical vocabulary of a field of study at an advanced level. For clinical terminology that is new to you, aim for concise, precise definitions. For theoretical terminology, which tends to be complex and multidimensional, leave a large space and make additions to your definition as your readings and discussions with others add to your understanding.

TYPES OF LITERATURE YOU WILL BE READING

Scholarly literature

Scholarly journals, articles and books go through a rigorous 'peer-review process' in which one or more experts on the topic review the material before it is accepted for publication. The authors are expert researchers with academic credentials (e.g., PhD), professional credentials (such as RN or MD), and institutional affiliations (such as a university or research institute). They write on narrow and specific topics related to research, theory, or practice in the health and social sciences. This literature is published by academic institutions (such as a university), organizations that perform original research (such as the WHO or CDC), and some commercial publishers (such as Sage). Within the scholarly literature, two important subsets are:

Review article: an article in a journal or a scholarly database that synthesizes all the literature on a topic in order to evaluate its overall strength and make recommendations for future research. These are helpful sources when you are looking for titles of scholarly articles to consult.

Systematic review: this is the term for a literature review that is focused on a single research question and tries to identify, evaluate and synthesize all the high quality research evidence relevant to the question. Many use a technique called 'meta-analysis', which is a statistical method of combining evidence. It has become essential for all professionals involved in the delivery of healthcare to know how to read and apply systematic reviews. Critics of systematic reviews, however, find that they are not always reliable and lack a universally agreed upon set of standards and guidelines. Nonetheless, they are essential sources. Perhaps the most widely used source of systematic reviews is *The Cochrane Database of Systematic Reviews*.

Grey literature

The name 'grey' has nothing to do with quality or colour. It is simply the name originally given by librarians to these materials to reflect the challenges of cataloguing them. The category includes reports, government documents, statistical reports, newsletters, bulletins, mission and policy statements, health promotion materials and fact sheets, among others. The authors include government agencies, research centres, universities, public institutions, non-profit organizations, and associations and societies. They are not published by commercial publishers. The purpose of grey literature is to provide scholars, professionals and lay readers alike with research summaries, facts, statistics, codes and standards, and other information related to the expertise of the publishing organization. Materials are written by experts within the publishing organization but often their names are not given. In these cases, the publishing organization is considered to be the author. (Indeed, it is not unusual for author, date and publishing information to be omitted altogether.) Examples of grey literature would include publications by the WHO, HMSO in the UK, the GPO in the US, the Queen's Printer in Canada, or the AGPS in Australia.

Primary vs. secondary literature

In social sciences and humanities, 'primary' refers to original source material that is closest to the person, period, or idea being studied. An example might be the personal papers of historical personages such as Florence Nightingale or Clara Barton. In these disciplines, 'secondary' refers to writings about the original sources. In medical and health sciences, however, 'primary' is used to mean peer-reviewed original research published in scientific and scholarly journals. 'Secondary' generally refers to review articles. As Nursing and allied health literature spans the social and medical sciences, you should be prepared to encounter the words with both meanings.

Professional literature

The purpose of this literature is to disseminate professional standards, news about the profession, professional trends, or editorial comment on the profession. It is written for an audience of professionals and practitioners within a field, and is written by experts on the topic with professional credentials and institutional affiliations. These materials may cite sources, but not as rigorously or as many as in the scholarly literature, and they may contain advertising. Examples would include the *Nursing and Midwifery Council Code* or the *Registered Nurse Journal*. These are important sources for codes, guidelines and practice standards.

STRATEGIES FOR THE WRITING PROCESS

A famous American architect once said that 'Form follows function'. His idea was that an architect should base the design of a building on the purpose or function it is being built to accomplish. This is as true of writing as it is of buildings. Each form of writing, or genre, has its own conventions and guiding principles around structure and use of language, depending on the purpose of the genre. Ultimately, our professional, academic and research purposes shape our writing practices, which in turn improve our ability to achieve those purposes.

To sum up, the form for any particular document is determined according to the reason for writing it. If the goal is to report on research, we write in a genre called 'research reporting' using the conventional structure known as IMRAD (Introduction, Methods, Results, Analysis, Discussion). If the goal is to promote healthy behaviours in the community, we use the genre of health education – materials such as brochures, posters, websites and social media. If the goal is to become reflective practitioners, we engage in reflective writing, and so on.

Broadly speaking, the writing process involves the following stages:

- defining the audience, purpose, and genre
- research and organizing/outlining
- drafting
- revising for accuracy and style
- preparing the presentation copy

Writing is an iterative process; in other words, it involves multiple repetitions of the same process. Each repetition is called an 'iteration' and the end-point of one iteration serves as the start of the next. The iterative process repeats until the desired goal is reached. In writing, the individual iterations combine reading, thinking, writing, and revising. The early iterations consist largely of reading and thinking, with some writing; the latter stages involve some supplementary reading but consist primarily of writing and revising. All iterations involve a lot of intense thinking.

Step 1: active reading and brainstorming

The first step in the writing process is active reading, which we talked about above. An additional important stage in active reading is 'brainstorming', a form of free associative writing in which you write down any and all thoughts that occur to you about your paper and the sources. Brainstorming can be done anywhere, even on public transport. Don't worry about quality – go for quantity. You can't know whether an idea will turn out to be useful or not, so just get it all down. If you typically suffer from writer's block at the sight of a blank computer screen or paper, you'll find brainstorming especially helpful. No longer will you be starting a draft with that paralyzing blank screen or paper in front of you.

Very important tip: Reading articles in this way is time-consuming and therefore can create stress. Unfortunately, you need to spend extra time learning how to read articles when you are in the early stages of a post-graduate programme. Don't despair – you will get faster at it as you build your knowledge base.

Step 2: do an outline

Whether you are a 'linear' or an 'organic' writer, never be tempted to skip the outline stage and jump into writing the draft. The outline is the skeleton of your paper – it's not something you can build in retroactively. A linear writer might prefer a detailed outline, while an organic writer might prefer a sketch of the main points. Whatever kind of outline you prefer, take the time to organize your thoughts and write one.

What does an outline do?

- keeps you on topic
- helps you avoid repetition of ideas or evidence
- allows you to check the logic of your argument
- allows you to see if you've addressed all the points you wanted to make
- it's an easy way to see if you've handled the topic adequately or need more points
- makes writing the draft much easier
- allows you to develop and refine your thesis (i.e., the central point you are trying to make)
- makes it easy to write an abstract or summary
- allows a supervisor/colleague/friend to comment and advise you on your work-in-progress

Step 3: write the draft

How you write your draft depends on whether you are a 'linear' writer or an 'organic' writer. Linear writers write a document from start to finish. They prefer not to leave a sentence or paragraph until they're comfortable that it's well written and makes its point. Organic writers will tackle whatever section they have something to say about at that moment. Maybe a lecture has sparked an idea, or they've found a new article they want to integrate as a source. They build their paper until most of it is written; then they shift to linear writing to make sure everything fits together.

It is an excellent strategy to set the draft aside once it is completed, for a few days or a week. Post-graduate students are frequently engaged in multiple pieces of writing at the same time, so this is usually easy to accomplish unless you are facing a looming deadline.

Step 4: revise and edit

To 'revise' means to 're-vision' – literally, to 're-see' at the **macro level** of overall content, organization, argument, and weight of supporting evidence.

To 'edit' means to sharpen or polish a document. Editing takes place systematically at the **micro level**. At the editing stage, you are attending to the details of language, format, and mechanics:

Use of language refers to word choice, tone, point of view and logical flow.

Format refers to the physical appearance and arrangement of the document – for example, margin size, font size, page numbering, tables and figures, and headings.

Mechanics refers to grammar, punctuation, syntax (sentence structure), spelling and lack of typographical errors.

Learning to edit your own work is such an important skill that is covered in depth in Chapter 5.

Step 5: proofreading

Proofreading the final copy is an important part of the writing process. It requires a lot of concentration and should not be left for, say, 3 a.m. when you are submitting the document at 9 a.m.

To 'proofread' means to ensure that the final, submitted version is completely free of any minor formatting and mechanical errors. It also means ensuring consistency in formatting and mechanics. Especially in long documents (such as a thesis), it is difficult to remember that on p.3 a numbered list was formatted using (1), whereas the numbered list on p.78 is formatted using 1).

Although some proofreading can be done on your electronic copy of the document, you will need to print out a hard copy to mark up, even if you will be submitting in electronic form.

The challenge in proofreading is maintaining a level of meticulous attention to detail, and keeping the mind focused on individual letters and marks rather than reading to follow the content. When we read, our eyes send a full set of data to the brain, but the brain acknowledges only enough of it to ensure understanding. The brain skips over the rest, where minor errors may be hiding. Here are some techniques that many writers find helpful to create the necessary focus:

- Each time you go through the document, read with a single purpose: spelling, punctuation, numbering, heading style, layout of tables and figures, or consistent use of key terms.
- Place a ruler beneath each line as you examine it to keep your eyes from skipping down the page.
- Move up the page from the bottom line to the top.
- Read the document from back to front.
- Read the document aloud to yourself or a colleague who is following a duplicate copy.
- Ask a colleague to proofread for you in exchange for proofreading something of theirs; proofread one final time when you get the paper back.
- Once you find an error or inconsistency in the hard copy, use the find-and-replace function of your electronic file to seek out all other instances of the error.

PROCRASTINATION, WRITER'S BLOCK AND OTHER BARRIERS

I speak with great authority on the subject of avoiding writing and then feeling blocked when I finally do get to it. If procrastination were an Olympic sport, I would bring home the gold for Canada.

It took me five games of solitaire on my computer to come up with those two sentences, and I am already considering what to make for dinner in three hours. Yet I have a publication record that, if not earth-shattering, is at least respectable. Clearly, then, there are ways to overcome the barriers that plague the lives of writers.

As with any other problem, identifying the source is the first step to finding a solution. Here are some of the main culprits:

Fatigue: When we go through periods of intense thinking and cognitive activity such as Masters or doctoral education requires, our brains respond in physical ways. The brain is plastic, meaning that particular activities done intensely and/or repetitively will cause changes in the network of neurons. The connections (synapses) between neurons change – new connections are made, existing ones are strengthened or weakened (or broken altogether). In other words, links between ideas are made stronger or weaker such that thinking of one thing will be more or less likely to draw along the other connected idea. This is why, after years of study and writing, our ability to think analytically and efficiently is improved. However, it also means that after individual sessions of study and writing, we may feel tired. The brain needs time to accommodate itself to the new architecture it has constructed and to absorb its new knowledge and ways of thinking.

The solution is simple: don't force yourself to keep writing. You'll just end up playing computer games or surfing the net. Instead, close the computer, stand up, and go do something else.

Time management issues: This problem can operate on two levels: the individual writing session and the overall writing plan. For the individual session, know how many hours you will work, how many breaks you will allow yourself, and what you will do during the breaks. The benefits of an overall writing plan are discussed in Chapter 1 but bear restating here: setting aside particular weeks or blocks of days for intensive writing sessions allows for mental preparation for writing and reduces the chance of distractions.

Distractions: By avoiding distractions, I do not mean you should lock yourself into a windowless room and chain yourself to the desk (perhaps with an intravenous coffee drip in your arm). The simple 'distractions' of a pleasant working space or music playing actually serve to foster creativity. Real distractions, however, rarely announce themselves as such. They present themselves as opportunities (such as extra paid work at a time of financial need) or responsibilities (such as a community council formed to fight closing of a local refugee centre) or obligations (such as a family member needing care or support) or promises made last year when your schedule this year was perfectly clear. The solution is to be as ruthless and selfish as you can be in refusing to take on new work, without utterly destroying precious relationships.

Don't know where to begin: If there are too many ideas swirling in a vague cloud in your head, you need to find a way to give them some structure you can work with. A simple mind map can be very helpful. Write an idea anywhere on a page and draw a balloon around it, then circle the central balloon with smaller balloons containing ideas or evidence related to the main one. Once your page is filled with balloons, draw a pathway of arrows between the major ideas, to show how one connects to another. From there, you can arrange the ideas as bullet points in linear order and use them as a writing outline. Do not feel, though, that you must follow the outline from start to finish when you write up the draft. The reader will read the final product that way, but you can write it in any order that feels comfortable.

Can't get started: Unlike a water tap, writing does not simply turn on. Plunking yourself down in front of the computer does not guarantee inspiration will flow. Many writers find it helpful to have a small set of rituals they perform in order to signal the brain that it is time to turn attention to writing. The rituals should not, however, be something that you can get too involved in, such as email or computer games. The goal is to empty the mind and create a writing environment. So, for example, the ritual could include making a cup of tea, tidying the desk surface from the previous day's work, and setting out the research materials you'll be using for that session.

Getting stuck: See above on fatigue. If you are stuck, it's probably a good idea to go do something else for a while, or take a physical activity break (e.g., do some stretching exercises, or a few yoga or tai chi moves, or go for a walk). If, however, you are stuck for more than two days, you are experiencing a block.

Writer's block: This is a form of intellectual paralysis in which no ideas or words come to you and when they do, they feel sadly deficient and terminally boring. The longer the block lasts, the more you feel it will never end. So, true to the definition that insanity means repeatedly doing the same thing but expecting a different result, you need to find a different way 'in' to the material. Helpful strategies include:

- Work on a different chapter or paper.
- Take a reading break and spend some time checking for new literature.
- Shift your way of thinking about your topic. For example, take the headings from your outline and write one each on index cards, then shuffle the index cards. Sorting your ideas in different ways can often reveal new perspectives and new ways to attack the material.

- Look a little deeper for the source of the block. Maybe this isn't writer's block at all. Maybe there is actually a problem developing with your research or theoretical direction and you need to confront it honestly. Sometimes we don't want to admit to ourselves that we need to change direction, with all the added work that involves. But until we do, we cannot move forward to the end-goal.

4

THE THESIS PROPOSAL

INTRODUCTION

Virtually every guide to writing a thesis, including this one, makes the point repeatedly that a long document such as a thesis must have a narrative arc. In other words, it has a central story line that unfolds from beginning to end. Without calling attention to itself, the narrative arc carries the reader along as inexorably as the plot of any action thriller. Perhaps not as thrilling, but just as consciously contrived and, in its own way, full of action.

Where do you begin to develop the narrative arc of your story? The answer is, right at the beginning, with the thesis proposal.

Many Masters and PhD students have commented to me that they found developing and writing the proposal more difficult than writing up the final thesis. At the doctoral level, the proposal stage is frequently a year long (or more), while writing up the thesis may be compressed into a few months as time-to-completion looms. Luckily, at that point you simply need to update and adapt the proposal and it forms the first chapters of the thesis. In addition, greater knowledge and skill meet up with deadline pressures to move you through to the end (plus, you may feel you've paid enough tuition, thank you).

At the doctoral level, developing and writing the proposal is an intense process that requires meetings with your supervisor (and, in North America, your committee), deep and comprehensive review of the literature, development of a research design and theoretical framework, building of research questions, and it very frequently involves applying for ethical approval. Passing the proposal stage is a major milestone, taken very seriously by the university, which will not pass the proposal unless there is confidence that the research it proposes can be done, and in a timely, ethical manner.

Typically, a thesis research proposal at both the Masters and doctoral level consists of three or four chapters (sections, in the case of the Masters proposal, but I will just use the word chapters for convenience):

1. Introduction (defining the problem: background and significance);
2. Literature review;
3. Theoretical review and framework;
4. Methods.

Depending on the topic, the two review chapters may be combined. Different institutions will have different policies and expectations, but 10–15 pages at the Masters level or 75 pages for a doctorate is a not unreasonable length.

DO THIS FIRST

In 2001, Prof. Janice L. Hewitt wrote a series of questions for post-graduate students at Rice University, in a handout called *Do This First*. Ever since, I have used these questions as a framework for advising students on how to begin writing their research proposals:

1. What, precisely, is the problem you are working to solve?
2. Why is that problem important?
3. What is the intellectual context of the problem? In other words, out of what previous work does your study grow? How will your research project differ from what has already been done?
4. What method(s) will you use to solve the problem?
5. What results do you expect?
6. What will be your unique contribution?
7. What are some possible applications of your work?

As Prof. Hewitt argues,

Once you have written the answers to those questions, you will have in mind the framework for your entire dissertation. As your research progresses, you will probably have to modify the answers, but that's to be expected. Being able to answer those questions precisely and concisely is still crucial. If you do that before you start writing, you will save yourself time and agony, I guarantee you. If you don't do it, you are likely to flounder around instead of writing a clear, persuasive narrative with a beginning, middle, and end.

I would add that your answers to these questions can be invaluable in initial meetings with your supervisor when you decide on a topic and a research approach. Taken together, the questions contain the entire narrative of your proposal. On a practical level, each answer forms the skeleton for a section of the proposal, as we'll see below. Equally important, they sharpen your focus at times when you may feel overwhelmed by the work and the writing of the proposal. They reassure you that you have a plan and you are accomplishing it.

The special role of the table of contents

It was difficult to decide where to discuss the table of contents because – although it is apparently humble and boring – the wise writer will return to it at numerous points in the thesis writing trajectory, where it can play an important organizational role. But as the proposal is the starting point of that trajectory, it made sense to mention the table of contents here.

The table of contents is more than a list of headings. It allows the reader to scan the entire content and organization of the proposal or thesis. It allows you as the writer to keep track of what you've done and still have to do. As the draft table of contents develops into the final one, it offers a great sense of accomplishment and excitement that the end is near.

The 'Do this first' answers will give you a preliminary table of contents that you can revise as you work on each chapter of your proposal or your thesis. Drafting a table of contents for each chapter as you begin it gives you an overview, as well as a division of labour that keeps the length of the whole from overwhelming you. Revising the table of contents when you finish a chapter lets you see that everything is there that should be – nothing left out but nothing duplicated – and in the most logical order. If something feels 'wrong' about the way your table of contents looks, pay attention and consider if you need to make changes in the chapter. If it feels wrong in the contents, it will feel wrong to the reader in the chapter itself.

FIRST CHAPTER: THE PROBLEM

Everything begins with Prof. Hewitt's first two 'Do this first' questions:

1.   What, precisely, is the problem you are working to solve?
2.   Why is that problem important?

The introductory chapter is structured to:

- define your problem; give background and overview
- provide a rationale: why, using support from the literature, do we need to look at this problem? What will doing so contribute to theory, research, and/or practice?
- identify the purpose of your study, i.e., your proposed focus on this topic

The objective of good health research is to improve wellbeing for many people. But any solution begins by isolating and identifying the problem. In other words, before you can get to the point of deciding on a research topic, you must begin big, with the problem. I use

problem here in a broad sense, not specific to some situation. For the specific situation, I use the word **need.** For example, a problem would be compromised patient safety. A need would be controlling medication errors in acute care settings. Narrowing further, a topic is the particular subject of study, its **purpose.** For example, a purpose might be to study the effect of modifying drug delivery systems on incidents of the most common medication errors in acute care settings, in order to improve patient safety.

To use the language of the *NHS Career Planner*, you may be interested in a career as a Clinical Academic, a Clinical Researcher, or an Academic Researcher, and the problem you will be interested in studying is to a large extent dependent on that career goal and the setting within which you intend to research or practise after getting the post-graduate degree.

SOURCES

NHS Career Planner, Summary of Level 9 Research. Available at: http://nursingcareers.nhsemployers.org/browse-segments/family-and-public-health/level-9-research.aspx

Hewitt, J.L. (2001) 'Do This First'. Unpublished instructional material prepared for use at Rice University, Houston, TX.

In discussions with your supervisor, here are some things to consider:

- Your personal and professional interests. This is an obvious consideration. You are going to be living with this project for a long time. If you don't have a passion for it when you start, it can quickly come to seem like a punishment. There is a warning here, however. Avoid topics that are too emotionally loaded for you, whether positively or negatively. If your feelings are too passionate, your goal too certain (e.g., to save all children from abuse because someone you know was abused), you can easily slip into researcher bias, where your bias affects the results or how you analyze them.

- Have you already been involved in research or in practice interventions and organizational change? Previous experience often shows us where our interests lie and also gives knowledge of what remains to be accomplished, what would be a new contribution.

- Supervisors may suggest possible topics based on the nature of their own research or on their wider knowledge of the gaps in knowledge and needs in the field. This is one of the most important reasons for careful choice of supervisor. If their research is of no interest to you, the topics or methodologies they propose will not be either.

- Do a broad review of the published research and grey literature to identify topics of interest and gaps in our current knowledge that you could fill. Reading the literature will also help you identify methodologies and theoretical frameworks you would be interested in pursuing. Don't hesitate to take advantage of the teaching resources offered by librarians, to help you learn to conduct your search.

- It is often suggested to look at the recommendations for future research in previous theses. But there is a warning here: people tend to move forward in their own careers based on their thesis research. This means they may have gone on to publish on their own recommendations, closing that door for you. If they haven't, it may be because the line of research didn't lead anywhere.

Ultimately, in deciding what to study, keep in mind that you would like to make an original, significant contribution to knowledge. At the doctoral level, this is a requirement (though not at the Masters level). As noted in Chapter 1, an original contribution does not mean a major clinical breakthrough or revolution in thinking. Progress in research is incremental and involves many members of the research community who build on previous research and dialogue with other researchers. Perhaps your research will do one of the following:

- apply an existing theory, model or research methodology to a new clinical setting
- rigorously test an intervention or assess a tool in a particular population
- extend previous research
- illuminate the lived patient experience with a particular illness in a new context
- fill a methodological gap in the way research in some area has been conducted
- conduct a scoping review to determine future research directions
- provide a new solution to an old practice problem
- integrate current theoretical perspectives to develop a new one

Defining the problem and its significance

Once you have a sense of the broad problem area you are interested in pursuing, answering these questions will help you build a story that will identify a researchable problem:

- What is the **nature** of the problem? (i.e., the discrepancy between what is and what should be)
- What is the **size and distribution** of the problem?
  - Who is affected?
  - Where are they?
- How **severe** is the problem?
  - How are people affected?
  - Since when have they been affected?
- What is the **context** of the problem? (i.e., the situation, events, or information that are related to the problem and that help us to understand it)
- Who perceives it as a problem?
- How urgent is the problem? What are the **consequences** if it is not resolved?
- What factors may have contributed to the problem?
  - What is the relationship between the problem and the **contributing factors**? Is it a cause-and-effect relationship or a mutual relationship

      (i.e., they co-exist and reinforce each other, for example, stigma about teenage abortion and secrecy surrounding it)

      o   Where do the contributing factors exist? In the community? Among healthcare providers? Within the healthcare system? Are they related to socioeconomic factors or social determinants of health?

- After identifying all the contributing factors, what factor **needs more investigation** in order for us to solve the problem?

The bolded words above are 'topic words', that is, the things that need to be talked about in the problem statement. It is particularly useful to position them at the beginnings of paragraphs, where they announce to the reader what the subject of the paragraph is. They build the flow of the storyline, moving from a description of the problem to its dimensions, to its causes, and finally to one part of the problem that particularly needs study.

SECOND CHAPTER[S]: THE LITERATURE REVIEW

This chapter (or two chapters, if the theoretical and research literatures are reviewed separately) answers the third 'Do this first' question:

3.   What is the intellectual context of the problem? In other words, out of what previous work does your study grow? How will your research project differ from what has already been done?

This chapter (or two) analyzes the research literature and the relevant theoretical perspectives. It should summarize the main research studies and theoretical frameworks; provide a rationale for using them (what are their strengths for your purposes); and provide a rationale for not using others (what are their weaknesses for your purposes).

    The narrative of the literature review presents the following argument to justify your proposed research: the problem has been studied for a particular length of time in these ways that demonstrate particular strengths and weaknesses, but none have solved a particular aspect of the problem, which my project will study in order to produce a better solution. The argument is somewhat comparable to the Darwinian struggle of life to identify a territory and then establish a niche within it that no other creature has successfully inhabited. Indeed, Swales and Feak (2000) use exactly this analogy to describe the way in which writers create a research 'space'. Researchers first 'establish a research territory … by showing that the general research area is important, central, interesting, problematic, or relevant in some way [and] by introducing and reviewing items of previous research in the area'. Then a niche is established 'by indicating a gap in the previous research, raising a question about it, or extending previous knowledge in some way'. Finally, the niche is occupied by outlining the purposes of the present research (Swales and Feak, 2000, p.175).

SOURCE

Swales, J.M. and Feak, C.B. (2000) *Academic Writing for Graduate Students: A course for nonnative speakers of English.* Ann Arbor, MI: University of Michigan Press.

The justification storyline answers these questions:

- How long has the problem been studied?
- What solutions have been tried in the past?
- How well have they worked?
- What is still missing?
- What future research is needed?

The justification narrative begins with an introduction that gives an overview of the literature and lays out the way you have organized the body of the review. For example, you might first look at the theoretical literature. Then you would discuss the empirical studies. (Or vice versa.) In the body of the chapter, it's not enough to go through the studies/articles one by one and just summarize them. That is the function of the annotated bibliography you have been building since the start of your programme. Now is the time to link them together in groups of related studies, with separate paragraphs on the ones that are most important. Move from strongest (or most often studied) to least. Briefly summarize each study, or grouping of studies, then evaluate it by describing its strengths and weaknesses, ending with what contribution it makes (or fails to make) to our current understanding of your topic. Overall, you want to leave the reader persuaded that a) there is previous research/theory that supports your investigating a problem and a related need, and b) there is a gap in the literature that your research is going to fill.

The narrative concludes with a summary of what you have just presented, and a concluding statement that ties the support/gaps in the literature to the purpose of your research. Once you have developed your research objectives and questions, they will also go here.

By the time you have completed your review, you will be in a position to decide whether the problem and need you have in mind can produce a feasible research topic, based on your judgement of the result of the review:

1. Sufficient high-quality research has been done
2. Some high-quality research but significant issues not covered
3. No or minimal high-quality research

If the answer is (1), it is time to change direction. Avoid the temptation to hang on to a topic you cannot make a new contribution to. Consult with your supervisor and if s/he agrees you need to find a new problem/topic, ask for some suggestions.

A research topic needs to be:

- relevant (e.g., to its broader problem, to advancing previous research)
- timely (i.e., is needed now)
- applicable (e.g., to clinical practice, to future research, to theory development)
- ethical, and
- not a duplication of previous research

Deciding on the theoretical framework

A framework is 'the abstract, theoretical basis for a study that enables the researcher to link the findings to nursing's body of knowledge. In quantitative research, the framework is a testable theory.... . A theory consists of an integrated set of defined concepts and relational statements that present a view of a phenomenon and can be used to describe, explain, predict, or control the phenomenon' (Burns and Grove, 1995, p.30). The theoretical framework plays an even more overt role in qualitative research, where theory affects the kind of information the researcher collects. Because research is not conducted within the controlled circumstances of quantitative research, qualitative researchers cannot simply collect everything: theory provides guidelines which allow these researchers to limit the kinds of data collected, and conceptual 'bins' to organize the data for interpretation.

The goal of the theoretical review is to provide:

- a summary of your main theoretical perspectives
- a rationale for using them (strengths)
- a rationale for what you will exclude (weaknesses)

As will be the case in the actual thesis, once the literature has been reviewed and a gap identified, you then formulate your research aims, objectives, questions, and/or hypotheses. However, the ability to narrow a topic to a researchable question (i.e., *what* to study) is bound up with decisions on methodology (i.e., *how* to study it), and so we move on here to discuss those decisions.

THIRD CHAPTER: METHODOLOGY

This section of the proposal addresses the fourth 'Do this first' question:

4. What method(s) will you use to solve the problem?

From a writing perspective, your task is to convince the reader that you intend to address your topic with a methodology that:

- is appropriate to answer the question[s]
- has an appropriate focus and scope
- considers and addresses any potential ethical issues
- has clearly defined boundaries so that the project can be completed in a reasonable length of time (i.e., 4–6 months of data collection).

The chapter is structured to describe and offer a rationale for the proposed

- research design
- sample and setting
- methods of measurement
- data collection and analysis process

In addition to arguing for and describing your methodology, a clear sense of planning needs to emerge in this section, so that the reader knows what is going to be done. For this reason, after the methodology is presented, the chapter does the following:

- presents a work plan and timeline for conducting the study (make sure you include plenty of time for the ethics review process if you will need to undertake this – see below);

- identifies the resources required and includes a budget;
- describes the background that makes you the 'right' researcher for this project, someone with the contacts needed to carry it out; and
- identifies a strategy for dissemination and utilization of research results.

A note on verb tenses: In a proposal, the Methods are written up in future tense, but in the actual thesis write-up you will use past tense.

CONCLUSION: THE CONTRIBUTION OF YOUR WORK

The concluding section answers the final 'Do this first' questions. It may conclude the Methodology chapter, or it may be its own chapter (though it will be shorter than the others):

5. What results do you expect?
6. What will be your unique contribution?
7. What are some possible applications of your work?

GETTING ETHICAL APPROVAL

If you thought you had already expended too much time and too many brain cells on administrative matters, welcome to the ethics review process. To gain ethical approval, you will need three skills:

1. the administrative skill to handle complex documentation and to submit it in advance of deadlines;
2. the writing skill to compress the content of the full research proposal in a way that compresses the narrative but in no way reduces its impact; and
3. a great deal of patience and planning.

History is littered with the victims of medical research, conducted sometimes with the best of intentions. As a result, all institutions within which research on humans is carried out have ethics review processes that are as rigorous and thorough as they can be. An international compilation of policies is provided by the Office for Human Research Protection, US Department of Health and Human Services (2010; cited in Egan-Lee et al., 2011, p.268). In Canada, policies and guidelines are set in compliance with the *Tri-Council Policy Statement: ethical conduct for research involving humans* (2010). And in the UK, the Department of Health's *Research Governance Framework for Health and Social Care* (DH, 2005) sets out the broad principles of good research governance. Based on each institution's local context, these foundational policies will be interpreted and applied. For this reason, you may need to go through more than one ethics review process – with the Research Ethics Board (REB) of your university and with the hospital or community agency setting where you intend to collect your data. Further, if you plan to conduct your study at multiple sites, each site will want to ensure that the research is safe and ethical for its patients or clients. It is impossible for a book such as this one to reflect all the complexities that can arise in a situation of such complicated policies and multi-layered processes. However, these tips will help you shoulder what can seem like a very heavy burden:

1. **Be informed.** Familiarize yourself with your own department's policies, timelines, and any guidelines for success they offer. This information may be available on the department website, but it is wise to consult personally with the department's research officer (or the equivalent) while you are deciding on your methodology. Also on the departmental level, some of the experienced research faculty may make available samples of their recent applications and REB responses for the benefit of novice researchers. Also, find out if your university's research office offers education sessions for novice researchers. Similarly, treat the university's REB as a resource. Request an initial consultation to familiarize yourself with the policies and processes, and follow up with another meeting when you are starting to develop your application. An REB consultant can offer you advice based on their experience with successful (or not) applications, or even offer solutions for the ethical issues you face. They may also be able to help streamline the process by, for example, communicating with other sites where you require ethical approval. In the case of a university and an affiliated teaching hospital, there may even be a mechanism that allows for a fully coordinated process.

2. **Be sure to allow enough time for a multi-stage process.** Because you cannot begin any part of your data collection until you receive final ethical approval, make sure you build enough time into the timeline of your proposal. Never assume that your initial proposal will be accepted as is, even if your research is low risk. Prior to beginning the REB process, your department may also have some sort of internal review process, which, although it adds time and work, is very helpful in identifying issues that may improve your application when it goes to the REB. For studies with minimal risks, especially at the Masters level, the institution[s] involved may allow an expedited process (also called a 'delegated' review). Normally, however, each review cycle (i.e., initial review or review of submissions) takes weeks. Consult the REB website or your contact there for the typical length of time. The initial review often necessitates modifications to your design, minor or major, and sometimes multiple resubmissions before final approval, especially for novice researchers. Even after final approval is received, you may need to re-apply for ethical approval (an 'amendment') if any changes occur as the project moves along (e.g., a change in study site or co-investigators).

3. **Be detailed and precise about your plans.** As Egan-Lee et al. (2011) point out, the REB will not be satisfied with general plans such as 'Interviews will be conducted until saturation is reached'. Instead, they will be looking for specific answers to very practical questions:

Who (e.g. who will have access to the data?), *what* (e.g. what areas of questioning will be used in the focus group?), *when* (e.g. when will audio files be deleted?), *where* (e.g. where will the data be stored?), *why* (e.g. why the specified number of follow up reminders are necessary during the recruitment phase) and *how* (e.g. how will participants be protected from possible coercion during the recruitment process. (pp.269–70)

The REB will also expect you to submit copies of all documentation related to the conduct of the study, such as recruitment posters, consent forms, and interview guides. They will also provide guidelines for the content and wording of this documentation. Not only should you follow them obsessively, but also be careful to be consistent in your wording across different sections of the application. These applications can be confusing and un-intuitive in structure.

4. **Be collaborative.** You may feel that the process of ethical approval is long and onerous, especially as the applications of novice researchers frequently require multiple, time-consuming revisions. You may even be worried about pressing issues such as an end to your grant funding if you can't get started on your data collection. But remember how important the goal of the review process is, and also remember that it is never in your interest to be impatient or demanding with the research officers who are working on your application.

FOR FURTHER READING

Burns, N. and Grove, S.K. (1995) *Understanding Nursing Research*. Philadelphia, PA: W.B. Saunders.

Canadian Institutes of Health Research, Natural Sciences and Engineering Research Council of Canada, and Social Sciences and Humanities Research Council of Canada (2010) *Tri-Council Policy Statement: Ethical conduct for research involving humans*, December 2010.

Department of Health (2005) *Research Governance Framework for Health and Social Care* (2nd edn). Retrieved from www.gov.uk/government/uploads/system/uploads/attachment_data/file/139565/dh_4122427.pdf

Egan-Lee, E., Freitag, S., Leblanc, V., Baker, L. and Reeves, S. (2011) 'Twelve tips for ethical approval for research in health professions education', *Medical Teacher*, 33: 268–72.

University of Toronto Office of Research and Innovation (2014) *Research Ethics and Protections: Humans in Research*. Retrieved from www.research.utoronto.ca/faculty-and-staff/research-ethics-and-protections/humans-in-research/

5

WRITING AND EDITING THE THESIS

OVERVIEW

- Managing a long document
- Revising your work
  - Tone and diction
  - Unity
  - Coherence
  - Emphasis
  - Paragraphing
- Editing your work
  - Clear writing
  - Concise writing
  - Precise writing
- An editing exercise

MANAGING A LONG DOCUMENT

For most post-graduate students, the thesis is the longest piece of writing they will do in their lives, unless they go on to write books. If you don't find writing it a daunting prospect, that may be because you are early enough in your programme to be in denial. The vast majority of students grow increasingly more apprehensive the closer the time comes when they will have to spend months writing their thesis. A few find the idea of writing a thesis so paralysing that they drop out of their programme.

Writing a thesis, though, is rather like building a house. There are thousands of small pieces that comprise rooms that comprise the whole. Similarly, a thesis revolves around a single research problem or question but has chapters that sequentially answer the questions in 'Do this first' (see p. 39). Within the chapters are sections with headings, each one a manageable chunk of only a few pages long. Like the hypothetical house, you have a blueprint and a need to get the thing built before the winter storms hit. All you have to do is follow the blueprint and you will succeed.

REVISING YOUR WORK

'Revising' and 'editing' are words whose meanings overlap in many ways and are often used synonymously. I am going to make a somewhat artificial distinction between them. I refer to 'revising' as reworking written material with a focus on macro-level issues of coherent flow of argument and larger decisions around language use, such as what overall tone to adopt. I use 'editing' in the sense of refining written material with a focus on finer issues of language use, in order to achieve:

a)   a writing style that is appropriate and pleasing in the academic context, and
b)   correctness in grammar, citation, punctuation and formatting.

At some point, everything you write needs to be revised and edited – that's obvious. But when should you do it? As you go along, crafting each idea, each sentence and paragraph before proceeding to the next? Or after the entire piece is drafted? Or perhaps in between, after a section is drafted? Writing handbooks often give sage advice on why one timepoint is better than another. But only you can decide which technique or combination of them works best for you.

Whenever you revise and edit, the result is always change and improvement in the text. Revising and editing have the benefit of slowing down the writing process and intensifying the thinking process. As you resolve even small issues of punctuation and wording, the larger context also grows clearer to you. Thus, at the same time as you build in 'correctness' and style, you also deepen and clarify your meaning and your argument.

Coming back to the analogy of a thesis as a house, the bricks of the thesis are the ideas and evidence; its mortar is the craft of your writing. Craft is the sum total of everything a writer does with language to engage the reader with the substance/argument of the writing. There is artistry to the craft of writing, but crafting language is primarily an objective process of multiple tasks and choices.

We make a distinction between the **content** and the **style** of a piece of writing. 'Content' refers to *what* is being said; 'style' refers to *how* it is said. Content is the information; everything that is part of the way the information is conveyed makes up the style. A great number of variables, including some intangibles, go together to make up what we call an academic writing style. Writing well in any style means making intelligent choices from amongst the alternatives language makes available to us. These include our choices about sentence structure, grammar, tone, diction, and even punctuation and verbs. To illustrate, these two passages convey the same content but in very different styles:

- While this may somewhat suggest the ineffectiveness of a passive approach to pain management for older adults, it does in no way promote the effectiveness of an active approach. This needs to be achieved through a review of the literature.

- A review of the literature suggests the effectiveness of an active approach to pain management for older adults.

The writer of the first passage no doubt believed it represents good academic style but the second passage is clearly better.

So what specifically constitutes good style in the academic context? First, there is a misconception (often the result of reading poorly written articles in academic journals) that academic style means using as many words as possible to say something, on the thought that this increases preciseness and clarity, or perhaps that quantity equals quality. As we see in the above examples, though, the wordiness actually makes the meaning less precise and less clear. Another misconception is that long words are better than short words in academic writing style. The 'long' words are in fact usually words of Greek or Latin origin and we'll see below that it isn't always good academic style to use them in preference to the 'short' words of Anglo-Saxon origin (though in medical sciences Latin-Greek words are frequently required). A final misconception is that academic style involves a lot of jargon. We'll see below that there is a difference between technical language and jargon, and that the latter is not desirable at all.

What, then, does constitute good academic style? In brief, it should be structured in a way that is appropriate to the particular genre of academic writing (in the case of a thesis, writing about research). It should also use the signals that the reader will be looking for, for example, signals that demonstrate familiarity with the literature, or that persuade the reader that there is an explanation for anything that could be perceived as a weakness in the research. Finally, good style uses the language and conventions that are used by the professionals in the field. Here we focus on editing to achieve the language and conventions that are expected in your thesis.

In the editing process, you might choose:

- to edit for all elements or correctness and style at the same time, moving line by line through the text to make changes on all levels
- to edit for one element only per read-through, increasing your ability to find all instances of one problem
- a combination: edit primarily for one element only, but make other minor corrections or circle/highlight/bracket other issues that will need some further thought, so that you can find them easily when you come to edit for that element.

Whichever strategy you use, editing is not accomplished on one go-through. No matter how many times you re-read your writing, you will find further corrections and changes to make. Only a deadline stops the process. Even when you write for publication, where multiple reviewers and editors read through the manuscript and you have several opportunities for corrections, it is always possible that you will find an error that everyone missed. My first significant publication was a dictionary – imagine my horror when I received my copies, hot off the press, and discovered a grammar error in the first sentence of the introduction.

The following sections explore the elements to focus on in the revision and editing process, moving from broader to narrower concerns:

Tone and diction

'Tone' refers to the intended emotional impact of a piece of writing. Writing can 'sound' neutral, angry, happy, intimate, concerned, or any other emotion. Notice that these two sentences, which convey the same information, have a very different tone:

> My patient had a supportive family which consisted of her husband and two adolescent children.

> I was amazed at the bond my patient shared with her loving husband and two teenage kids.

We convey tone through word choice. In writing, 'diction' refers to the specific word choices made by the writer to establish a particular tone. (In speaking, 'diction' has a different meaning: it refers to clarity of speech.) We speak of diction as being formal, informal, or colloquial.

Another thing that we need to understand about tone and diction has to do with the history of English. English has two root languages. Prior to the year 1066, Anglo-Saxon was a Germanic language, so different from modern English that it is hardly recognizable as English on first encounter. In 1066, the Normans successfully invaded Britain, and French (a Latin-based language) became the language of the ruling classes. That, combined with the Church's introduction of Latin and Greek as the languages of scholarship and religion, had a profound impact on the English we speak today. It means, among other things, that we often have choices of words to express the same meaning, one derived from Anglo-Saxon and one from Latin or Greek. For reasons that likely have to do with the social history of the two root languages, words of Latin and Greek origin are considered to be more formal and objective in tone. Informal or colloquial diction tends to draw on Anglo-Saxon origins (as do our ripest swear words).

The language of medical sciences, by which we describe the composition and mechanistic functioning of the human body, is not a natural language like English. No baby's first words were ever 'myocardial infarction'. It is a technical language that has been constructed over the past 600 or so years by snipping together bits of Latin and Greek that 'unpack' for the healthcare professional into very specific information about what has happened [infarct = break] and where [cardio = heart]. It is rigorously precise, unlike the lay term 'heart attack', which inaccurately suggests an external force 'attacking' the heart like a thief in the night.

It is a mistake to think that writing in formal academic or scientific style means always choosing Latinate diction. Given the complexity of the technical terms of science and medicine, it is usually preferable to seek simpler word choices for other elements in your sentences, both to highlight those important terms and to maintain forward movement. Writing that is overly Latinate is lifeless and challenging for the reader. The title of an excellent short article on the importance of achieving a clear and engaging writing style says it all: 'What can make scientific papers extremely heavy going is the daunting and lifeless quality of their prose' (Dixon, 1993).

Table 5.1   Levels of diction

Formal	Informal	Colloquial
conducted	did	
examined	looked at	eyed
completed	finished	over with
serendipitous	fortunate	good luck

Table 5.2   Latin versus Anglo-Saxon diction

Latin origin	Anglo-Saxon origin
approximately	about
additional	more
conduct	do
demonstrate	show
necessitate	need
obtain	get
provide	give
solicit	ask for
sufficient	enough
utilize	use

SOURCE

Dixon, B. (1993) 'What can make scientific papers extremely heavy going is the daunting and lifeless quality of their prose', *The Chronicle of Higher Education*, 21 April: Sect. B:5.

There are, however, certain conventions around the use of verbs in research writing that prefer Latinate words – we saw some of them above in Tables 5.1 and 5.2. For example, in research writing, 'conducted' is preferred to 'did' or 'was done', and 'examined' or 'explored' is preferred to 'looked at'.

Writers are often told to 'avoid medical jargon' in their writing, but what exactly is jargon? For healthcare professionals, medical language is simply a language they have been trained in, what we call the 'common discourse' of the health professions. It is only when highly technical medical language is used for a wider audience, without explanation or without a need for it, that it becomes jargon. This is why it is used liberally when, for example, writing an article related to a pathophysiological process, but not in designing interview questions for participants from the community.

Unity

Every unit of a thesis, whether a sentence, paragraph, section, or chapter, must give the readers a sense of unity. That is, each unit should centre on one subject that is announced near the beginning, and everything in it should contribute to a description or understanding of the subject. If unity is present at all these levels, the thesis itself, inevitably, will achieve unity. It is easy, in the flow of drafting, to veer off into interesting but ultimately irrelevant ideas or evidence. The result is confusion for the reader, who loses the thread of your argument. As you revise, be on the lookout for digressions – sentences, paragraphs, or even sections that just don't 'fit' – and be ruthless about expunging them. It is very difficult to cut out material that you a) like very much and/or b) spent a lot of time writing, but you must force yourself. I myself never delete the material completely. Instead, I move it into a file labelled 'Good Bits' and go on fishing expeditions in the file whenever I start a new writing project, to see if there is something I can now use.

Coherence

The parts of a sentence, paragraph, section, chapter, or whole thesis need to relate clearly to each other and be logically ordered. The material needs to be organized in such a way that it tells a story: the first sentence/paragraph/section tells us what we are talking about, then the rest of the paragraph/chapter/thesis tells us its story. The story can be developed a number of different ways, such as chronologically (e.g., the steps of designing and conducting a research study; the history of policy development), positive to negative or vice versa (e.g., the strengths/weaknesses of a study or body of literature), most to least important or vice versa (e.g., study results; impacts of social determinants of health), question[s] to answer[s], and others.

What holds the story together is 'structural coherence', that is, the use of language to signal particular types of relationships among the parts:

Repetition: As writers, we are intimately familiar with what we are trying to say, and we may sometimes feel that we are boring our readers if we are too repetitive. But in fact, repetition of key words and concepts is an integral part of establishing coherence in argument. For example, it is typical at the beginning of the Methods chapter to restate the research question.

In an effort to introduce variety by seeking synonyms for key words, writers can unwittingly introduce confusion for the reader, caused by the fact that synonyms are only sometimes truly synonymous. Often there are subtle differences in meaning; for example, if a key concept is 'empathy', switching at times to 'sympathy' breaks the flow – they aren't the same, and coherence is interrupted as the reader wonders if a new concept has been introduced.

Logical connectors are transitional words and phrases that create logical relationships such as addition, contrast and causation. Table 5.3 classifies the main logical relationships and gives you a variety of synonymous terms to choose from.

Table 5.3   Connecting words and phrases that create coherence

To show addition	To compare	To contrast	To give an example	To emphasize
a second point	also	although	for example	above all
again	by comparison	but	for instance	certainly
and	equally	conversely	in fact	chiefly
also	in the same manner	however	in particular	especially
another	in the same way	in contrast	namely	indeed
as well	likewise	by contrast	particularly	in fact
besides	similarly	nevertheless	specifically	in particular
first, second …	than	nonetheless	such as	more importantly
for one thing … for another		on the contrary	that is	most importantly

To show addition	To compare	To contrast	To give an example	To emphasize
further		on the other hand	to illustrate	primarily
furthermore		rather	as an illustration	unquestionably
in addition		still		
moreover		though		
next		unlike		
or/nor		whereas		
too		yet		

To restate a point	To summarize or conclude	To indicate logical relationship	To introduce a qualification or concession
again	in conclusion	as a result	admittedly
in brief	in other words	consequently	after all
in effect	in short	for this reason	all the same
in other words	in summary	if ... then	despite
in short	that is	since	even if
in simpler terms	therefore	so	even though
that is	to sum up	therefore	frequently
to put it another way		thus	generally
to repeat			in a sense
			in general
			in spite of
			occasionally
			usually
			while it is true that

Signposts appear at the beginning of a paragraph, section or chapter. They tell the reader what to expect and they often pose a question or introduce a theme that the forthcoming section, paragraph or chapter is going to explore. Signposts tell readers where they are on the narrative arc of your thesis or chapter. Examples include:

- The following section presents ...
- This literature review is structured as follows ...
- Following a description of the six agencies that serve the Greater London Area, this chapter analyzes ...

Frames indicate the beginning and ending of a section or chapter. On the chapter level, framing devices take the form of short paragraphs, one at the beginning to lay out the chapter's structure and one at the end to summarize the contents and/or argument of the chapter. For sections, framing devices include sentence structures such as these:

- First, ... Finally, ...
- To begin with, ... To conclude, ...

Focusing highlights and reinforces key points. For example,

> As mentioned earlier, …
>
> The central issue is …
>
> It must be stressed that …

Emphasis

In speech, the audience is able to understand what the speaker wishes to emphasize through his or her words, through changes in pitch, inflection and volume, and through body language and gestures. The writer has no such tools – words are all we have.

Anyone who has ever taught courses and marked student writing has at least one story of a student who petitioned for a higher mark on the argument that she or he did in fact include elements that the marker claimed were missing. The student then points triumphantly to a single sentence buried at an apparently random spot within the paper. The marker's response is that there was no way of knowing that s/he was supposed to focus on that sentence. There was no sense of emphasis.

Here are some of the ways we establish emphasis in writing:

1. Emphasis through positioning:

In this respect, writing and verbal communication are the same: the most emphatic positions are first and last. This principle is true on any level of writing: the sentence, paragraph, section, or whole document. Generally, we expect the beginning to establish the topic, and the ending to present the new idea about it. For example, I might say:

> Poverty is a risk factor for premature morbidity.
>
> One risk factor for premature morbidity is poverty.

They are both clear, informative sentences about poverty as a social determinant of health, but they establish different points of view. The first sentence emphasizes the topic of poverty; the second emphasizes the topic of risk factors for premature morbidity.

2. Emphasis through independent clauses:

An independent clause is a group of words that can stand by itself as a sentence. In other words, it contains at least one subject and one verb that indicates an action or state. A dependent (or 'subordinate') clause, on the other hand, cannot stand by itself. Although it contains a subject and a verb, like an independent clause, it depends on another clause (an independent one) for its meaning. As a result, an independent clause is more emphatic than a dependent clause. Thus, if one idea is more important than the other, make the less important one into a subordinate clause. Compare these two examples. The first uses two independent clauses and the reader is left to assume they are of equal importance. In the second, the dependent clause is not only completed by the independent clause but the word 'although' also announces the relationship of contrast between the two.

> This conflict is managed by nurses on a daily basis and it can cause emotional dissonance.
>
> Although it is managed by nurses on a daily basis, this conflict can cause emotional dissonance.

3. Emphasis through modifiers:

These draw attention to the most important part of a sentence. Notice how emphasis changes in this example from Bell (1995), depending on where the word 'only' is positioned:

[Only] one subject [only] remembered [only] the medication [only] in the morning

4. Emphasis through typography:

Typography is used in moderation in academic style to create emphasis, for example, by bolding or italicizing the names of themes that emerge from interviews in qualitative research. Writing in all CAPITAL letters is not done.

5. Emphasis through sentence length:

Short sentences are more emphatic than long ones, as long as the writing contains a variety of sentence lengths. If every sentence is a short one, the sense of emphasis is quickly lost and the writing feels immature. Uniformly long sentences also destroy any sense of emphasis, and are both cumbersome and boring. When there is a variety of sentence lengths, not only is the writing style most interesting, but the shorter sentences take on an added 'punch'.

SOURCE

Bell, L. (1995) *Effective Writing: A guide for health professionals*. Toronto: Copp-Clark.

Paragraphing

A paragraph is a group of sentences relating to the same idea or topic. There is no correct length for a paragraph, although there are common misconceptions that it must not extend past a certain number of words, lines or sentences. However, a transitional paragraph can be as short as one sentence. On the other hand, a substantive paragraph can extend to a page or even more. Generally, however, when a paragraph exceeds a page (double-spaced), you should question whether it covers only one topic, or whether it should be split. As you revise your paragraphs for unity, coherence and emphasis, keep in mind the type of paragraph each one is and make sure that it is fulfilling its function:

An **introductory** paragraph describes:

- the main topic or idea of the paper or section it introduces
- the extent or limits of coverage
- how the topic will be developed
- the writer's approach to the topic.

A **body** (substantive) paragraph:

- develops one idea and its supporting evidence
- contributes the substance of ideas and information. Most paragraphs are substantive: they develop the argument and deliver the evidence

- there is no 'correct' length for a substantive paragraph but they are usually three sentences or more but less than a double-spaced page.

A **transitional** (non-substantive) paragraph:

- provides a bridge from one section of a paper to another.
- may be as short as only one sentence
- ties together what the reader has read so far and what is to come
- can be positioned as the concluding paragraph of a section and offer a brief summary of the section
- can also be positioned as the introductory paragraph of a new section and offer a preview of its structure and argument
- does not contribute any substance to the argument, but functions to move the argument forward.

A **concluding** paragraph:

- briefly restates the main points of the section or chapter
- often moves the reader to consider upcoming sections or chapters, or may make recommendations.

EDITING YOUR WORK

Clear writing

We say that a text is clear if a competent reader who knows the meanings of any technical terms used will understand it on the first reading in the way the writer intended.

Writing can be **unclear**. Unclear passages are challenging and frustrating for readers as they try to figure out what you mean. Here's an example:

> Explanations concerning why cardiovascular training may be beneficial in allevia-tion of some of the manifestations of FM syndrome include activation of the endog-enous opiate system which may function in the modulation of pain (Davis, 2007), physical exercise has been shown to improve mental state (Kerr, 2010), and may pro-vide a sense of purpose and control over a person's body, and provide some resistance of trained muscle to microtrauma (Tremblay, 2008).

There are two clarity problems in this long sentence. The first is word choices that are unclear. 'Explanation' is not a very precise word, ranging in meaning from a verbal expla-nation to the answers to research questions provided by scientific studies. In this case, 'studies' is what is meant. Second is the structure of the sentence. The reader must work through four different grammatical structures. This clarity problem can occur when we need to include a great deal of information in a sentence. Here, it's a list of the benefits of exercise for improving pain management, mental state, and physical conditioning. For maximum clarity in complex sentences, an effective strategy is to use 'parallel construc-tion', that is, use identical structures to introduce each item in the list. In this case, the little phrase 'on the' will do the job:

✓ A number of studies have examined the benefits of cardiovascular training in alleviating some manifestations of FM syndrome, specifically, **on the function of** the endogenous opiate system in the modulation of pain (McCain, 1996), **on the role of** physical exercise in improving mental state (Kerr, 2010), **and on the resistance of** trained muscle to microtrauma (Tremblay, 2008).

Writing can be unclear if it is **overly formal.** Trying for 'academic English' can lead to sentences that are dense and difficult to read, but not very informative. They are full of unnecessary words and awkward passive verb constructions. The wish may be to achieve a formal, elegant writing style, but the result is a lifeless writing style that seems to take forever to make its point:

✗ While this may somewhat suggest the ineffectiveness of a passive approach to pain management, it does in no way promote the effectiveness of an active approach. This needs to be achieved through a review of the research literature.

✓ A review of the research literature suggests the effectiveness of an active approach to pain management.

Writing can be **ambiguous**. Ambiguous writing offers at least two different valid interpretations:

The biologists discussed redoing the experiment for three days.

Which way did you take the meaning of this sentence? That perhaps the biologists sat in a coffee shop for three days to discuss redoing the experiment? Or that they'd originally done a two-day experiment and were considering making it longer? Or both? The problem here has to do with what we call 'positioning'. In other words, you should place words or ideas that are related to each other as physically close to each other as possible. By placing the 'three days' beside either the authors or the experiment, we link it to whichever one we want:

✓ For three days the biologists discussed redoing the experiment.

✓ The biologists discussed taking three days to redo the experiment.

Concise writing

I have made this letter longer than usual because I lacked the time to make it short. (Blaise Pascal, *Lettres provinciales*, letter 16, 1657)

Conciseness is a high information-to-words ratio in a text. The opposite of conciseness is wordiness. A concise sentence is not necessarily a short one. Conciseness means using exactly the appropriate number of words, whether that is five or 50. But let's start with a short sentence that demonstrates the point perfectly:

It is certain that needs will increase.

Here we have seven words. If we highlight the words that express a meaning, we have:

It is **certain** that **needs will increase**. ('will' is included because it is part of the verb)

'It is' and 'that' don't convey any meaning, so why include them? Depending on whether we'd like to emphasize the certainty or the needs, we can rewrite in these ways:

✓ Certainly, needs will increase.

✓ Needs will certainly increase.

If you remove three meaningless words out of every sentence in a ten-page paper, you will have fewer than eight pages, and it will be a much clearer paper.

The opposite of conciseness is wordiness, where we use words that repeat what other words already say, or where we simply use more words than are necessary:

✗ A large number of athletes practise some type of a warm-up activity prior to exercising. The goal of warming-up is to prepare the athlete physiologically and psychologically for exercise.

✓ Many athletes warm up to prepare physically and mentally for exercise.

Table 5.4   Wordiness versus conciseness

Original	Revision
a large number of athletes	many athletes
practise some type of a warm-up activity prior to exercising	warm up
the goal of warming-up is to prepare the athlete	to prepare
physiologically and psychologically	physically and mentally

Here is a list of common wordy phrases along with shorter ways to express the same meaning:

a number of	several
appears to be	seems
at the present time	now
at the same time as	while
at this/that point in time	now/then
conducted a study that looked at	studied
due to the fact that	because
for the reason that	because
if conditions are such that	if
in a timely manner	promptly
it is often the case that	often
of a large size	large
on condition that	if
prior to the present time	ago
utilize, utilization	use
was variable	varied
were responsible for	caused

Finally, omit altogether wordy phrases or sentences that fulfil no useful purpose, such as these:

It is evident that this term is associated with much ambiguity. Many concepts and ideas come to mind upon first hearing this phrase; however, a true grasp of its meaning is quite difficult to establish.

In this connection the statement can be made that …

It is a fact that …

It is emphasized that …

It is interesting to note that …

Precise writing

Precision refers to being exact rather than vague, and specific rather than general:

- ✗ The profits of No-Name Pharmaceuticals rose dramatically last year.
- ✓ The profits of No-Name Pharmaceuticals increased 13% in fiscal 2014.
- ✗ This paper examines pain management techniques for our rapidly aging population.
- ✓ This paper examines pain management techniques in elder-care institutions in three urban UK settings.

Avoid unnecessary qualifiers:

- ✗ This paper **attempts to explore** the relationship between harm reduction initiatives and rates of homelessness in Vancouver.

Why be hesitant? You are exploring, not just trying to.

- ✓ This paper **explores** the relationship between harm reduction initiatives and rates of homelessness in Vancouver.

Use specific numbers and percentages:

- ✗ Almost half of the participants were drawn from a single setting.
- ✓ Forty-eight percent of the participants were drawn from a single setting.
- ✗ In this study, coaches sometimes reported that their athletes use visual imagery to prepare for competition.
- ✓ In this study, 20% of coaches reported that their athletes use visual imagery to prepare for competition.

Be careful that potentially vague words like 'significant', 'important', 'meaningful', 'unique' are used precisely. 'Unique', for example, means 'the only one of its kind'. It does not have degrees:

- ✗ Smith's study uses the most unique approach our public health nurses had ever seen.
- ✓ Smith's study uses an approach previously unknown to our public health nurses.

If something is 'important' or 'interesting', we must know to whom it's important or interesting, and specifically why:

✓ Smith's (2005) findings on carious lesions in childhood (<5 yrs.) will be important for public health nurses working in agencies that serve low income clients.

Avoid vague words such as 'good' that have no precise meaning. Also avoid intensifiers like 'very', 'really', 'actually'. They add nothing to the meaning of the sentence:

✗ Tracheal intubation is **actually** the best method of securing the upper airway.

✓ Tracheal intubation is the best method of securing the upper airway.

Avoid useless words like 'exist'. If it didn't exist, you couldn't write about it.

✗ There **exists** a large body of literature to support this suctioning technique.

✓ A large body of literature supports this suctioning technique.

AN EDITING EXERCISE

When it comes to strength-training exercises such as push-ups and bench presses, the more repetitions you do, the better you get. This is equally true of revising and editing. Practice does indeed count toward perfection, especially as you grow aware of your own patterns of poor or incorrect writing. You may be too busy with your own writing to practise with the exercise below, but if you can find the time, it is very helpful to edit writing that is not your own. This is because it is much easier to see what is and is not working in someone else's work than in your own. See what you can do to improve the following piece of writing in all the dimensions that we discussed above. One possible revision is given at the end, but there is no right or wrong – you may prefer the version you come up with!

Original version

There is a relationship between characteristics of the social environment and health that much recent research is focusing on in the UK and around the world. There was a study done of the British civil service in London in 1990 by Smith and Black which reveals very noteworthy differences in mortality for most causes of death between four classes of male civil servants. From 1985–1990, which was the five year period studied, the male civil servants who were in the lowest grade died at three times the rate the civil servants in the highest grade did.

The findings of the study were all the more noteworthy for the reason that none of the employees were living in poverty. Furthermore, all the employees had good job security. They all worked in the same city of London. Finally, none of them were ever exposed to industrial hazards of any sort during the period of the study.

The most interesting gap between the mortality rates of the highest and lowest classes were for respiratory diseases like, for example, lung cancer and chronic bronchitis, which are all related to smoking. The amount and extent of smoking was really different between the civil service grades. Smith and Black showed in their study that 29 per cent of the top grade civil servants smoked, which was compared by the authors to 68 per cent of the bottom grade. It is important to note, however, that the authors also found in their study that lower grade civil servants who were non-smoking had higher death rates due to chronic heart diseases than their higher grade counterparts did.

Another study done in Britain found that the organization of work and in particular the freedom to make decisions are the basis for the strong link between social class and heart disease. After they reviewed international research thoroughly and effectively, they found that when the 'decision latitude' at work is lower, the proportion of smokers found is higher. They looked at the links between social class and chronic heart disease on an international level and they considered the evidence from the civil service study, and then they attested that: 'above a threshold of poverty, position on the social hierarchy per se may be a more important determinant of health and disease than material condition.'

-381 words

Revised version

Recent international research has focused on the relationship between characteristics of the social environment and health. Smith and Black's (1990) study of the British civil service in London revealed significant differences in mortality for most causes of death in four grades of male civil servants. During the study period (1985–1990), all participants enjoyed similar material conditions: none was living in poverty; all had good job security; all lived in London; and none were exposed to industrial hazards. However, the male civil servants in the lowest grade died at three times the rate of those in the highest grade. The largest gap between the mortality rates of the highest and lowest grades was for smoking-related respiratory diseases like lung cancer and chronic bronchitis: 21 per cent compared to 61 per cent. Significantly, only 29 per cent of the highest grade smoked, compared to 68 per cent of the lowest grade.

Another British study (Taylor et al., 2000) reviewed international research, including Smith and Black (1990), and found that when the 'decision latitude' at work is lower, the proportion of smokers found is higher. The authors concluded that the organization of work and in particular the freedom to make decisions are the basis for a strong link between social class and disease; that is, above a threshold of poverty, position on the social hierarchy may be a more important determinant of health than material condition.

-229 words

WRITING THE INTRODUCTION CHAPTER

OVERVIEW

- Structure
- Background: defining the problem and its significance
- Reviewing current approaches
- The study purpose and contribution
- Final note: overviews, summaries, and where to include them

STRUCTURE

The Introduction begins the narrative arc of the thesis by fulfilling two essential functions: it introduces the problem, its significance and the purpose of the study, and it gives an overview of the organization of the thesis. Especially in a qualitative or mixed-methods study, or in a publication thesis, it is also likely to contain some reflective element. It is not typically a long chapter, though it can be, and there is a variety of ways to divide it up, depending on what you want to prioritize in terms of depth and detail, and your larger purpose.

Of the six dissertation models used in this book (see pp.3–4 for full titles and brief description), three include a reflexive section in the first chapter, in which the writer 'locates' her or himself as a person, professional, and researcher. For example, JL's narrative inquiry weaves 'scientific discourse … together with narrative writing and poetry' (p.2), allowing her 'to engage both the scientific and the artistic aspects of self' (p.3) and the technological in heart surgery. It is only appropriate, then, that she chooses to devote her first chapter to a 'Prologue', a 14-page personal reflection on the relationship of art and science in general and in her own life experience in particular. It is her second chapter that lays out her problem, etc. Similarly, MRV begins his first chapter with a six-page reflection on the genesis of his research and his location as an 'insider' in the South Asian community.

Because it follows a very conventional pattern, FWM is used as the primary model in this chapter.

BACKGROUND: DEFINING THE PROBLEM AND ITS SIGNIFICANCE

The chapter may begin with a very brief (one paragraph) overview of the thesis, or may jump directly into the background. The background section needs to: a) define the problem and its significance; b) summarize our current approaches to the problem in order to identify a research need; and c) state the purpose and benefits of the study.

Chapter 4 laid out a number of questions to help in developing your problem for the research proposal. Using the key words from those questions in your write-up will ensure that the reader is clearly given all the relevant elements: the nature of the problem, its size and distribution (who is affected and where they are), severity (how and since when have they been affected), context (social, medical, etc.), consequences, contributing factors, and factors that need more investigation. This list is intended to be helpful, not prescriptive, and requires your own decisions. For example, in discussing the severity of the problem of hypertension in pregnancy, FWM does not need to address the question of 'since when' because we can assume there have always been pregnant women with hypertension.

Broadly speaking, arguments follow one of two patterns of movement: from a general statement to a specific one, or from a specific statement to a more general one. Of the two, moving from general to specific is the more common pattern, and particularly useful to introduce the problem, as we see in FWM's first two sentences:

> [1] Hypertensive disorders occur in approximately ten percent of all pregnancies, and are identified as a significant health issue (WHO, 1988). [2] Hypertension in pregnancy is associated with fetal/infant morbidity and mortality and is a leading cause of maternal death in Canada (Health Canada, 2000). (p.1)

[1] introduces the two most important words in the problem ('hypertensive', 'pregnancy') and describes the problem as 'worldwide', emphasizing that the prestigious WHO is concerned. [2] identifies what the health issue is and narrows the focus to Canada.

REVIEWING CURRENT APPROACHES

This section of the chapter is the reader's first introduction to the knowledge base that will be reviewed in detail in the literature review chapter[s]. Unlike that detailed exploration, this section only briefly summarizes the approaches that have been pursued in order to solve the problem and why these approaches have not yet solved it. The object is to demonstrate the merits of the approach you wish to follow and the limits of others. A great deal of qualification is used in this section (qualification and the reasons for using it are discussed on pp.102–3). FWM, for example, summarizes three approaches to managing hypertension in pregnant women: the two conventional approaches of clinical management and drug therapy (antihypertensive medication) and the psychophysiological approach she intends to test. Her language and phrasing emphasize both the widespread use and the limits/risks of the conventional approaches. In the following examples, the qualifiers are bolded and logical connectors are in italics:

> **Although** hypertensive disorders in pregnancy have different etiologies, with diagnosis either predating or occurring during the pregnancy, clinical management **tends to be** similar ... (p.1)

> Measures ... used outside of pregnancy to reduce hypertension **are not recommended** in hypertensive pregnancy, **due to inadequate evidence** of their benefit for this population group. Current recommendations for clinical management of hypertension in pregnancy **are limited**: ... (p.1)

> *However*, as **there are concerns** about potential fetal risks in association with antihypertensive medication use, pharmacological approaches to management of hypertension in pregnancy **may not be desirable**. *Therefore*, **other less potentially harmful** approaches to blood pressure reduction **have appeal** ... [p.2]

On the other hand, when she discusses the psychophysiological approach, she emphasizes its relative newness and potential benefits. The qualifiers are bolded:

> Psychophysiological therapies ... have been used **successfully** in reducing blood

> pressure in non-pregnant adults, **although** the study of guided imagery as a single therapy has been **quite limited**. (p.3)

> ... the simple and inexpensive strategy of guided imagery provides a **reasonable** therapy to test ... (p.3)

> Medline and PsycInfo database searches for 1975 to 2004 revealed **only** two published evaluations ... (p.4)

FWM concludes her rationale for studying guided imagery by logically connecting her arguments about the three approaches:

> [1] The evidence that psychophysiological therapy may reduce blood pressure, the current lack of useful clinical approaches to the problem of hypertension in pregnancy, and concerns about antihypertensive medication [2] all pointed to the need for a controlled evaluation of the effectiveness and feasibility of guided imagery for blood pressure management in hypertensive pregnant women.

[1] Each of the three approaches is briefly summarized in the first half of the sentence. [2] The second half of the sentence links the state of current knowledge to a rationale for why the study is needed. The phrase 'all pointed to the need' emphasizes the strength of her conclusion. The word 'controlled' points forward to the RCT design. The phrase 'guided imagery for blood pressure management' points forward to the purpose and objectives, which follow immediately after, in her next paragraph.

THE STUDY PURPOSE AND CONTRIBUTION

The Introduction chapter concludes with a statement of purpose that is generated logically from the problem. It tells the reader in a clear, concise statement what the specific goal or aim of the study is, in terms of addressing or elucidating the problem. The purpose is often called goal[s], aim[s], or objective[s], but for convenience I use the term 'purpose'. Sometimes the research questions are also given here, rather than at the end of the literature review chapter[s].

The statement of purpose needs to follow logically from the first two sections. In FWM's chapter, the first section established hypertension in pregnancy as the problem, the second section reviewed the current approaches managing it, and now she transitions into her purpose and objectives:

> The primary purpose of this pilot RCT was to provide preliminary indicators of the effects of guided imagery compared to a quiet rest intervention on a) blood pressure and b) anxiety. Additional objectives were … (FWM, p.5)

The purpose states the RCT research design, with two words (pilot, preliminary) that emphasize the groundbreaking nature of the research. The statement of the purpose also includes three PICO elements: **Intervention** (imagery), **Comparison** (to rest) and **Outcomes** (blood pressure and anxiety). An improvement would be to add the final PICO element, **Population** (in hypertensive pregnant women).

Another important element in this concluding section is an explanation of the potential benefits of the study, its significance and contribution. This is the first of several positions within the thesis where the contribution of the research is highlighted, and it typically comes just before or after the statement of purpose. For example, KE's subsection titled 'Significance of the Study' summarizes what her study is expected to contribute to retaining nurses in acute care settings, and ends this way:

> **Nurse leaders can use** the information to improve their practices **and organizations can use** the information to plan leadership development and support programs. (KE, p.7)

FINAL NOTE: OVERVIEWS, SUMMARIES, AND WHERE TO INCLUDE THEM

It is important to make the organization of the thesis transparent to the reader by including overviews (looking ahead to a new section) or summaries (wrapping up what has just been said) at strategic points. There are a number of reasons behind this convention: a) overviews and summaries link the parts of the thesis narrative, forming transitions from one to the next; b) the thesis is a long document and the readers are not intimately familiar with it the way the writer is, so these are helpful signposts; and c) the practice follows a general convention in all research reporting to accommodate readers who read only sections of articles and who therefore need signposts to orient what they are reading to the larger article. Some thesis writers rigorously include overviews and summaries, not just for every chapter but for every section of every chapter. However, there are certain positions where they are almost always included:

1. in the first chapter, often at the end, an overview of the entire thesis
2. an overview at the beginning of each chapter and a summary at the end
3. very commonly at the beginning and end of the sections within chapters

Beyond that, if you feel the need for an overview or summary to create a transition between sections, include one. It is probably better to overdo them and be asked to cut some than it is to get feedback from an examiner who is confused about how the thesis progresses.

Overviews and summaries serve the important functions of linking the narrative and orienting the reader, but they do not make for exciting prose. They are clear descriptive writing and use simple, direct sentences; for example, 'This thesis reports on a research study that …'.

MRV concludes his first chapter with an extensive thesis overview, which begins this way:

> The thesis has eight chapters. The second chapter provides a literature review. Chapter three presents the methodology and methods I adopted for this study. The following chapters four, five and six present the findings of the study. Chapter seven presents discussion and chapter eight concludes the thesis. Below I outline the structure of the thesis. (p.20)

He then devotes one paragraph to each chapter in order to outline it.

7

SEARCHING AND EVALUATING THE LITERATURE

OVERVIEW

- Purpose and argument of a comprehensive review
- Searching the literature
  - Step number one: get to know the librarians
  - The search process
  - The value of tracking citations
- Evaluating quantitative (QN) and qualitative (QL) research
- The parts of a quantitative research article and what to look for
- The parts of a qualitative research article and what to look for

PURPOSE AND ARGUMENT OF A COMPREHENSIVE REVIEW

Universities place tremendous emphasis on literature review, at every stage from the undergraduate dissertation in UK (and some North American) pre-registration Nursing programmes to the PhD and publication. Everything has a substantial section of literature review. Why? A good part of the answer lies in the model of evidence-based practice.

In 1991, Gordon Guyatt, one of a group of doctors working at McMaster University's school of medicine in Canada, coined the phrase 'evidence-based medicine' to describe medical diagnoses based on the best research and clinical evidence available (Van Rijn, 2007). Like many great breakthroughs, it seems an obvious approach once someone had thought of it. But until the approach was developed, health professionals relied on past practice and consensus; further, new practices took a great deal of time to spread and become universally adopted. Evidence-based medicine, and by extension evidence-based practice, is based on the principle that evidence takes precedence over consensus. As Dr Brian Haynes, chair of the department of clinical epidemiology and biostatistics at

McMaster said, it 'is an attempt to ensure that the evidence is coming from research that is properly valued – not overvalued or undervalued – and that that evidence doesn't have to wait 20 years for implementation' (Van Rijn, 2007).

The comprehensive literature review demonstrates your ability to find all the relevant material, and it demonstrates your ability to evaluate what you find.

What are the main barriers to good literature review?

a. inability to sift through volumes of material
b. inability to evaluate as opposed to describe
c. inability to link the material reviewed to your own research purpose or your own investigation of a problem or issue
d. under- or over-estimating the amount of literature you need to search and evaluate

In the health professions, when we speak of the literature, we mean everything that has been written on a health topic by accredited scholars and researchers.

A 'literature review' or 'critical review' is a classification and evaluation of the literature, organized according to a guiding concept or topic. This could be a research question, a search for the best evidence-based practice, or an understanding of a problem/issue within health. 'Critical' in this sense does not mean seeking out the negative; it means to evaluate something based on both its strengths and weaknesses and come to conclusions about its usefulness for understanding or solving the problem at hand.

Literature review tells us both what has and what hasn't been accomplished in an area of study. Think of scientific progress and our understanding of the human experience as stretching on a time line from prehistory to the stars. Literature review shows us where we are on the line – what we know (or think we know) and what we still hope to discover.

The ability to review the literature critically is important for a number of reasons. First, to become an expert in any field of endeavour, you must comprehensively know your field. Literature review develops two crucial skills which develop that knowledge:

• the ability to find the literature on a topic, and
• the ability to read, understand and evaluate it.

Researchers conduct reviews of the literature to justify proposed studies, to uncover patterns of findings in the field, to enter into scientific or professional debate, and to discover gaps in knowledge that lead to future research questions. Research reviews are often the first step toward making scientific discoveries and social interventions in our society.

In addition, critical reviews of state-of-the-art literature permit the health professional to make informed decisions, to practise in an expert manner, and to influence policy in his or her field. We should make a distinction here between making a decision and solving a problem. Problem-solving refers to situations in which there is one right answer that can be determined and applied; in contrast, decision-making involves tradeoffs among alternatives. Critical review helps us weigh the available alternatives and synthesize them into best practice or policy.

To conclude, a good literature review is not just a summary, but a critical evaluation and synthesis. The best critical appraisals are:

1. organized around and directly related to the topic they explore;
2. a summary of what is and is *not* known about the topic within the literature;

3. able to identify areas of controversy and problem;
4. able to identify future directions for research, practice, policy, or theory.

When one enters post-graduate studies, especially after years in a professional career, the research literature may feel flat, in the sense that it all seems of equal quality. There is a tendency to assume that the quality is high. After all, how could it get published otherwise? Alas, the answer is that sometimes poor or marginal articles do get published. Having said that, even the highest quality research has limitations, either within its design and/or conduct, or in terms of its usefulness for your topic. Finding and articulating those limitations within a review is not done for the sake of being negatively critical – it is done as a way of understanding how and where we should be moving forward.

SOURCE

Van Rijn, N. (2007, January 6). Medical journal hails Canadian 'eureka moment'. *Toronto Star*, p.A3.

SEARCHING THE LITERATURE

Step number one: get to know the librarians

Success in post-graduate studies depends on access to scholarly resources. So step number one is to get to know your university's library system and what it can do to support you. (Ideally, an investigation of the library resources would have been part of your decision to apply to your programme of post-graduate studies in the first place.) There are two parts to what you need to know: information about the library itself, and the scope of what the librarians do.

The library

The size and quality of a university's collections, both print and digital, contribute to a university's reputation as a research institution. Research libraries around the world are ranked by the prestigious Association of College & Research Libraries (ACRL), a division of the American Library Association. Rankings are determined based on statistical analysis of 300+ performance indicators, including size of circulation and reference holdings, total staff, circulation and reference transactions, and total library expenditures. In North America, for example, the highest ranked research libraries are Harvard, Yale and the University of Toronto. The library website or – better yet – a visit to the library itself can give you useful information on the following:

- What is the size of all collections and specifically the ones related to your field?
- What is the reach of the library services, including borrowing and lending from other institutions around the world?
- What level of technological resources does the library offer, both onsite and on its website?
- How do librarians support your discipline? What level of collaboration and participation exists between the library and your faculty/department?

The librarians

Librarians as a profession are smart, dedicated people who use their available resources to the fullest in order to support the learning and research of faculty and staff of a university. The key word here is 'available'. A first-rate, well-funded research university will invest heavily in its library system. Even when institutions are not well funded, it says a lot about them if they make the choice to devote scarce resources to the library system. In an ideal environment, librarians are able to offer you help that includes the following:

Tours and workshops to orient new students to their information services

Tutorials and reference services on:

- the library's information services
- navigating the library catalogue
- searching specific databases such as Medline or CINAHL
- reference management software such as Endnote, Refworks or others
- copyright practices and where to go for additional information
- scholarly communications information sessions: what are your options for publishing and how to identify models that best suit your publishing needs
- university initiatives on digital repositories for thesis, dissertations and research data
- information technology tools applied to education, research, and access
- non-traditional sources of information and where to find them
- archives – what they do and where to find them

Consultations

Are librarians available to help you if you have problems with your search or questions on how to conduct it? By online chats? By telephone? By appointment in person?

If you have problems with your search, or questions on how to conduct it, your librarians will offer some or all of the following consultation services:

- One-on-one consultations
- In-person, email and/or chat quick reference
- Online forums
- Workshops on
  - basic, advanced, and non-traditional sources of information
  - keeping current
  - citation management
  - scholarly communications
- Specialized (medical/health/science) focused and multidisciplinary workshops
- Video tutorials and screencasts

The search process

New post-graduate students begin with search engines they are already familiar with, such as Google Scholar. Gradually, they learn to become comfortable navigating discipline specific databases such as MEDLINE and CINAHL and other academic databases, as well as finding grey literature. Their searches grow yet more sophisticated as they seek out not just the mainstream of scholarly thought but also alternative and contradictory positions.

This chapter does not go into detail on the mechanics of searching electronic databases because information technology improves so rapidly that anything said here will soon be out of date. But the strategy of searching is independent of the technology we use to accomplish it, whether we use the index cards of pre-computer libraries or the vast databases of today's information technology systems. The search process for a thesis literature review follows these steps:

1. Break research questions into searchable concepts
2. Determine which databases to search, and why
3. Understand what search filters are and where to find them
4. Use grey literature to complement your search
5. Document and store the material you find.

SOURCE

Gerstein Science Information Centre (2013) Systematic Reviews [Webpage]. Retrieved from http://guides.library.utoronto.ca/systematicreviews

Your librarians will be able to offer you resources – online, in workshops, or in person – to teach you how to perform these steps. To help you get started, it's helpful to have a brief guide to the landscape you will be exploring. As part of its online guide to *Nursing e-Resources for students conducting reviews for thesis/dissertation or coursework*, the Gerstein Science Information Centre describes some of the top medical, scientific and allied health databases for Nursing research:

CINAHL

CINAHL is the Cumulative Index for Nursing and Allied Health. It contains fundamental content for nursing and other allied health professions, such as physical and rehabilitation therapy. Some of this content cannot be found in PubMed or MEDLINE. CINAHL matches terms to Subject Headings in the same manner as MEDLINE.

MEDLINE

Premier database for biomedical journal articles. Interface allows for expert searching (e.g., use of MeSH) when conducting systematic reviews, scoping reviews, etc. Covers approximately 4000 journals; international in scope.

PsycInfo

Major database for scholarly literature in psychology and behavioural sciences. Covers approximately 1800 journals as well as books, reports, theses and dissertations.

EMBASE

Large biomedical database with emphasis on drug research and pharmacology; good coverage of alternative therapies, occupational therapy and physical therapy. Covers approximately 4000 journals (1200 of which are not in MEDLINE); international in scope.

PubMed

Provides free access to MEDLINE. Includes additional selected life sciences journals not in MEDLINE.

Cochrane

Systematic reviews of the effects of healthcare interventions. Also contains the Cochrane Central Register for Controlled Trials (CENTRAL) and the Database of Abstracts of Reviews of Effects (DARE).

HealthSTAR

Articles about health services, technology, administration, and research. It focuses on both the clinical and non-clinical aspects of healthcare delivery.

BIOSIS

Large medical database which also covers agricultural sciences, botany, biotechnology, zoology and biology in the broadest sense. Covers thousands of journals as well as conference proceedings. Good for supplementing a search that deals with plant or animal organisms (e.g., bedbugs).

SCOPUS

Scopus is a major multidisciplinary database for the social sciences, life sciences, health sciences, physical sciences, and arts and humanities. Scopus covers research literature published in academic journals, Open Access journals, conference proceedings, trade publications and book series. Scopus also covers 200 million quality Web sources, including 12.7 million patents.

Web of Science

A major multidisciplinary database. Web of Science consists of the Arts & Humanities Citation Index, the Science Citation Index and the Social Sciences Citation Index. It can be searched as a database in the usual manner, but you can also obliquely search the citation indexes for articles that cite a known author or work.

Health and Psychosocial Instruments - HAPI

Provides access to information on measurement instruments (i.e., questionnaires, interview schedules, checklists, index measures, coding schemes/manuals, rating scales, and more) in the health fields, psychosocial sciences, organizational behaviour, and library and information science.

SOURCE

Ayala, A.P. and Gerstein Science Information Centre. (2013, 3 June) Nursing
  e-Resources [Webpage]. Retrieved from http://guides.library.utoronto.ca/
  content.php?pid=243652&sid=3172615

The value of tracking citations

The process of searching the literature also involves identifying key citations in sources
and tracing the cited authors and others from reference lists in order to locate other
sources. Tracking citations among articles is an extremely efficient way of learning the
scope of research on a topic across time, methodologies, and results. One American
doctoral student interviewed by Green and Macauley (2007), for example, reported on
the multiple tasks accomplished within the tracking process:

> I run database searches and then I find articles that look potentially germane … .
> Then I make notations on them, and when I get a group that seem to be pretty good,
> I'm also collecting the bibliographies from some articles and looking to see what
> authors are mentioned commonly or most often. (p.324)

SOURCE

Green, R. and Macauley, P. (2007) 'Doctoral students' engagement with
  information: 'An American-Australian perspective'. *Libraries and the
  Academy* 7(3), 317–32.

EVALUATING QUANTITATIVE (QN) AND QUALITATIVE (QL) RESEARCH

Research is a systematic investigation to establish facts, principles or generalizable knowledge. When we critique a study, we examine the system the researchers use (its design); the
methods they use; how they analyze what they find; and the facts, principles or knowledge
they claim to have established.

   The two broad categories of research, quantitative and qualitative (also called traditional and interpretative) are abbreviated here as QN and QL. Increasingly, researchers
conduct mixed-methods studies that combine the two. For example, someone who is studying nursing issues in neuroscience and trauma might investigate a particular cognitive
consequence of traumatic brain injury, but also interview patients about the impact it has
had on their ability to conduct their daily lives.

Quantitative research designs

- experimental and quasi-experimental
- correlational
- observational

- case study
- survey
- developmental

Qualitative research designs

- ethnography
- hermeneutics
- phenomenology
- grounded theory
- narrative
- arts-based
- action

QN research uses the scientific method to discover knowledge of the body as a diseased versus an undiseased organism. In this fundamental way it differs from QL research, which seeks knowledge of the body as a lived experience, and seeks to understand the social, psychological and behavioural aspects of health and healthcare. The purpose of QN research is to arrive at an understanding of the world by describing and explaining phenomena through established principles for scientific research. What, it asks, causes disease in the body? What can we apply to the diseased body so that the effect is a restoration of the undiseased body? QN research is hypothesis-driven; in other words, researchers predict what will happen if they conduct a test or experiment in a controlled setting. Then they conduct their research and conclude whether the results support (or don't) their prediction.

QN research breaks down situations it seeks to study into key aspects called 'variables', which simply means the thing the researchers are going to change (called the independent variable) and the things they hope will change as a result (called the dependent variables). In medical and nursing research, the independent variable is often referred to as a 'risk factor'. The researchers perform a treatment or procedure that manipulates the independent variable in some way[s], observe and record what happens to the dependent variables, and then measure and statistically analyze these results (also called 'findings') in order to draw their conclusions.

For example, researchers might hypothesize that the independent variable of yoga has an influence (called a 'correlation') on the dependent variable of stress among pregnant women. They will then perform a study on two equivalent groups of pregnant women: first they measure the 'baseline' levels of stress in both groups. Then one group (the 'experimental' or 'intervention' group) receives a 'dose' of yoga classes over a certain period of time; the other (called the 'control' group) does not. Then they repeat the stress measurements and compare the dependent variable of stress between the two groups to see if there is any correlation to yoga, i.e., if the yoga has influenced a greater change in stress levels than no yoga.

We said earlier that QN research studies the diseased body, while QL research seeks knowledge of the body as a lived experience, or the 'lived body'. Qualitative studies seek an in-depth understanding of human behaviour (*how* we behave) and the reasons for it (*why* we make our decisions to behave certain ways). They explore how we experience both health and illness, and the many factors outside the pathophysiological process which impact that experience, such as our family and social supports, our socioeconomic level and educational background, our cultural/racial identities, and other social determinants of health. These are all variables within our lives that cannot be controlled in the same way that QN researchers control their variables. QN research collects data in numeric form and manipulates it statistically. QL research collects data in words and images, then teases out its meaning in a variety of analytical ways. Thus, qualitative researchers identify and formulate research topics from different perspectives and use very different methods of collection and analysis than quantitative researchers.

A final and very important difference between the two lies in their assumptions about the role of the researcher. In QN research, the researcher attempts to be an objective observer and to control or remove any impact (or 'bias') he or she might exert on the research process. In QL research, however, the assumption is that the best way to learn about a situation is to participate in it. Thus, the researcher is acknowledged as an active participant in the research process, sometimes in active collaboration with the participants.

Both types of research are important, and each has its drawbacks. With its reliance on fixed methods of collecting data, such as scales and questionnaires, quantitative research captures only the data that fits those pre-set limits and thus may misrepresent the complexities of the disease/illness process. Qualitative research, on the other hand, sometimes focuses too closely on individual results derived from small samples and is not easily used to make connections to larger groups of people or situations. As well, because the researcher plays an active role in the research, there is always the risk that the researcher's individual beliefs and values may over-influence his or her data collection and analysis.

THE PARTS OF A QUANTITATIVE RESEARCH ARTICLE AND WHAT TO LOOK FOR

IMRAD or IMRD are the common abbreviations for the standard sections within published research studies: Introduction, Methods, Results, (Analysis), Discussion. QN research strives for 'rigour'. A rigorously conducted study:

- has a tightly controlled design;
- uses methods that can be verified and repeated by other scientists;
- has precise measurement tools; and
- studies a sample that accurately represents the larger population of interest, so that the study results can be 'generalized' to the whole population.

What follows is a description of the sections you can expect to find in an article reporting on a quantitative study, although you will encounter variations of this structure. There are also questions and comments to guide you in judging the strengths and weaknesses of these studies as you critique them.

Title

A good title summarizes, as specifically as possible, what the study is researching. Does it do that? For example, 'Pain management for Wales' aging population' is far less informative than 'Pain management techniques for chronic arthritis in five long-term care settings in Wales'.

Authors and their affiliations

Who are the authors of the study? What institutions and/or universities are they affiliated with? Does it seem to you that their qualifications and affiliations make them suitable people to be studying the topic? You can also look up or link to other articles they've written; that will give you a sense of their experience in their area of expertise. Looking briefly at their other work will also help you understand their current study more easily, as researchers frequently work on related topics over a number of studies.

Abstract

An abstract is a brief summary, which condenses in itself the argument and all the essential information of a paper. You don't need to comment on the abstract in your critique, but reading the abstract gives you a good overall understanding of the article and makes it easier to follow.

Introduction

Background: The first thing the authors do is give background on the problem they are studying. For example, in a study on pain and chronic illness, the authors might outline the rising rates of chronic illness and the health risks of long-term use of common painkillers.

Significance and relevance of the problem: The authors should tell you who is affected by this problem and how. They should tell you why it is important that we solve it. What will happen if it isn't resolved? What if it is?

Statement of the purpose: The purpose of a study is generated from the problem. It tells us in a clear, concise statement what the specific goal or aim of the study is to address or study the problem.

Brief literature review: It is important for researchers to position their research on the timeline of our knowledge about the problem. In order for us to understand the need for their research, they need to give us a clear and concise summary of what previous research has and has not established, what its strengths and limitations are, and what the gap is that the current study seeks to fill.

Research purpose, aims, goals, objectives, questions, and/or hypotheses

Researchers will include some (but not likely all) of these. Although different in some important ways, they all have the same intent, which is to make clear, concise statements that identify and describe the reasons for conducting the study, what exactly it will study, and how the researchers are going to study it.

A research purpose, goal or aim identifies and describes the change to the problem the researchers hope will result from their study. For example, a study might have the following aim:

> To evaluate the nutrient intake of Finnish pregnant women and relate it to the use of vitamin/mineral supplements.

A research objective is more specific: it identifies and describes the independent and dependent variables that will be studied to address the problem. For example, an objective might be:

To measure nutrient intake adequacy of vitamin/mineral supplement users and non-users among Finnish pregnant women.

More specific still, a research question is an interrogative statement that the researchers develop to direct their study. For example:

What is the nutrient intake adequacy of Finnish pregnant women who use vitamin/mineral supplements compared to non-users?

Method

Study design: This refers to the method the authors use to carry out their study. Broadly speaking, there are two types of design in QN research: experimental and descriptive. In an experimental design, a treatment or intervention is given to one randomly selected group of participants and not given to another randomly selected group of participants (the 'control'). The control group has carefully defined characteristics that are equivalent to those of the treatment group. Researchers also control factors that go beyond the participants alone: they will establish controls to prevent any other variables from influencing the results – for example, they might exclude participants with medical conditions in addition to the one they are studying. This design, called a randomized control trial (RCT), is the most robust one for establishing cause-and-effect relationships, and it is considered the 'gold standard' of research designs.

Quasi-experimental designs do not randomize their participants into treatment and control groups. They are used when it isn't ethically possible to have a control group – for example, if you are studying a life-saving surgery, you cannot withhold the surgery from one group of patients. Or it may not be practically possible to have a control group, for example, when researchers want to assess whether some intervention that is currently being used has made a difference since it was first initiated. These researchers might use case histories and chart reviews rather than current patients in what is called a retrospective design. For example, if we want to know if a particular smoking cessation campaign instituted ten years ago has worked, we could look at lung cancer rates in a geographic area where the campaign took place compared to one where it didn't. But even if the rates are lower, we can't claim to have proved the campaign caused the effect of lower rates because we have no way of controlling variables that have occurred in the past. Nonetheless, quasi-experimental designs make a very important contribution by enhancing internal validity when randomization is not possible.

Whether experimental or quasi-experimental, the authors should describe the following aspects of their design:

- Do they identify independent, dependent and other research variables?
- Do the researchers identify extraneous or confounding variables? These are variables that could distort the effects of the independent variable or that cannot be controlled by the researchers (either because they weren't anticipated or because they emerged only after the study started).

Description of the sample and setting

'Sample' refers to the subset of the population that has been selected for study. For example, rather than studying all Finnish pregnant women, researchers will recruit a number of individuals whose demographic characteristics (age, socioeconomic status, education level, and others) make them representative of that larger population. 'Sampling' refers to the process of selecting the sample. Look for these things:

- Who was eligible to be included in their study (inclusion criteria) and who was not (exclusion criteria)?
- How and where did they find the people who were eligible, and is it clear why they found them that way?
- Did they give a letter or form to inform potential participants about the study and get their 'informed consent' to participate? Do they tell you their research was approved by an ethics review board or some other ethics approval process? Researchers have an ethical obligation to protect the wellbeing of their participants; to do no harm; and to protect confidentiality and privacy. In other words, they should treat human participants as they would be treated, and treat animal subjects humanely.
- How large was their sample? Do they explain how they know that sample was large enough to produce usable results?
- How many participants are there at the beginning compared to the end? Do they account for any participants who left the study before it was completed (called 'sample mortality')?
- How many groups are there and how many in each group? The numbers should be equivalent – if they aren't, do the authors tell you why?
- If the balance of males and females among the participants seems important to you, based on what they are studying, do they make an attempt to balance the numbers?

The setting refers to where the study is conducted. Settings can be natural, partially controlled or highly controlled. It should be clear to you why they chose this setting, and how they controlled it (if they needed to).

Methods of measurement

Researchers should describe the 'instruments' they used to measure their study variables. These may be scales and questionnaires, physiologic measurements, and/or observations.

- Do they describe the instrument[s] they are using to measure their study variable? Do they say who developed it? If the authors developed it themselves, they should describe their development process.
- Do they describe how they know their instrument is both reliable and valid for measuring what it is supposed to measure? 'Reliability' refers to the extent to which it measures consistently. 'Validity' refers to the degree with which it measures accurately.

Data collection process

They will then describe how they performed the tests, measurements, etc., on the participants. If it was necessary for researchers or participants to be 'blind', they should describe how they did this. If the researchers themselves didn't collect the data, they should describe how those people were trained.

Results

Results sections describe what they found, that is, the data they collected. We expect to learn how the authors analyzed the data they collected and what results they obtained to answer their research questions.

Data analysis procedures

In quantitative research, statistical methods are used to analyze the data. Statistics can help to determine if the relationships between independent and dependent variables are due to chance or due to the effect of the treatment (i.e., cause and effect). Unless you have taken a course in statistics, you will find these sections hard to follow. The word to look for is 'significance'. Significance in this context does not have the common meaning of 'importance'. Instead, it is a specific term – a significant result is one that is unlikely to have occurred by chance.

Presentation of results

Results are presented in the same order as the research questions or hypotheses, and are given from most important to least important, or strongest to weakest. The text should give the important information, with tables and figures to provide full details.

Discussion

The purpose of this section is to interpret the results in order to answer their research question[s] or support the hypotheses. Discussion sections interpret the results to make points. For example, a results section might say:

> In the treatment group, 116 (84%) participants reported improvements in functional ability.

The discussion section might then say:

> The unexpectedly high percentage (84%) of participants who reported improvements in functional ability suggests that this pain management technique, although controversial, is highly effective in older adults with arthritis.

The section should discuss the results in the same order they were presented in the results section.

Relationship to previous literature

The argument of this sub-section runs as follows: (1) here are the ways in which our study is similar to previous studies – this supports what we found. (2) Here are the ways in which our results are different from previous studies: (a) either their study or ours was flawed, incomplete, or simply different in some way; (b) we've identified the causes of the differences and they don't matter. Finally, the authors argue that: (3) our results advance our previous knowledge on the problem in these ways.

Identification of the limitations

No study is perfect – it isn't possible. So it's important for the authors who, after all, know their study best, to identify what the weaknesses in their study were. They will also identify any ways in which future studies could overcome or improve them.

Conclusions

This section completes the train of argument that ran from the results (here's what we found) to the discussion (here's the relationship between what we found and the question we asked) by adding conclusions (here's what we can conclude about our research problem and the larger population our results can be generalized to). The authors should also do the following:

Identification of implications for the field

The authors should describe any larger purposes for research, policy, theory or practice that this study contributes to. They need to convince us that their study has added to our current body of knowledge.

Recommendations for future research

This may be its own sub-section or be combined with a description of the study's strengths and limitations. They may suggest that future research make changes in methodology, or they may suggest new research questions or new populations for study.

References

Their references are an excellent resource for you, an easy way to discover what the current and important literature is on this research area. You will also get a sense of who the major researchers and theorists are as you read multiple articles and see the same sources cited in many of them.

Acknowledgements

Academic and scientific journals have ethics guidelines that require authors to acknowledge their funding sources and any possible conflicts of interest. For example, there has been a number of high-profile cases in which it was revealed that researchers had been funded by pharmaceutical companies to test their drugs, and then published results that were falsely positive or which omitted negative findings or side effects.

THE PARTS OF A QUALITATIVE RESEARCH ARTICLE AND WHAT TO LOOK FOR

Like QN research, QL also strives for 'rigour' but in different ways. It strives for 'trust-worthiness' in interpretations of the data. One of the great challenges of QL research lies in finding a practical tool for assessing it. In an important article on evaluating qualitative health research, Eakin and Mykhalovskiy (2003) note that quantitative health research derives from the work of clinical epidemiologists in developing evidence-based medicine. For this reason, they argue, quantitative checklists like the one in the last section focus on *how* the research is conducted; that is, they focus on 'procedure'. As Eakin and Mykhalovskiy put it, quality is judged 'on the basis of the researcher having made the right choice of method and having executed it in the right way' (p.190). As QL researchers attempt to capture in language the richness and fluidity of human life and health, however, their methods also need to be flexible and diverse. Their methods become resources for engaging with and understanding the topic of inquiry and their findings. These methods resist the standardization that makes QN research so much easier to checklist. Instead, Eakin and Mykhalovskiy advocate focusing our evaluative energy on the analytic content of the research, its 'substantive' offering, that is, what the authors actually say about the phenomena they have investigated and how they relate their research practices to their findings (p.191).

Unfortunately, the dominant stream within health research was historically (and still remains) QN. In addition, the world of healthcare management is a very pragmatic place and QL research is often not generalizable to larger populations or intended to propose solutions to immediate problems. For these reasons and others that have to do with the publication process, the appraisal of QL research is usually done using templates derived from QN checklists. A good example of this is the widely used Critical Appraisal Skills Programme (CASP) checklist for qualitative studies (available at www.casp-uk.net/).

Because of the publication process, many QL researchers structure their articles and use language that is consistent with the widely used checklists. Thus, the questions proposed below to help you evaluate QL studies draw from traditional checklists but also focus on the substantive aspects of QL research. The goal is: a) to help you explore how the different elements of the research contribute to the authors' ability to derive meaning from their findings; and b) to help you use the research to improve your practice and advocate for your patients.

Introductory material

- Do the authors introduce their study with the background, significance, and relevance of the topic they are studying?
- Do they identify a purpose for their study?

The research question

- Does the research question provide a 'positioning device' for understanding the nature of the investigation and its findings? Does it feel like a good starting point?
- Does it identify and describe the kinds of knowledge the researchers were seeking in/through the research process?
- If their research question[s] changed through the process of conducting the research, do the authors tell you how, when and why?

The researcher[s]

Unlike the objectivity and 'view from outside' that is expected of QN researchers, in QL the researchers are assumed to be subjective – otherwise they wouldn't be able to engage with their participants and develop a 'view from inside'. Thus, it's very important for them to tell us about some of the following things at least:

- Do the researchers tell you anything about themselves? Any personal background? How they came to be interested in researching this topic?
- Do they describe any aspects of their 'social location'? Social location refers to the position we occupy within our society. That position is determined by our gender, age, class, income, education, family and social network, among others. When researchers consider their social location, it helps both them and us to understand how all these factors will affect the way they engage with their research and the ways they interpret it. It's especially important if they are studying a society that is not the one they belong to. Unfortunately, it is generally the case that researchers in developed countries have greater resources for travelling to developing countries to conduct research than the opposite.
- Did they engage in any self-reflexive process? Do you get the sense that it allowed them to approach their research with creativity and sensitivity?
- Can you identify their theoretical or conceptual 'location'? In other words, what kinds of theory shape their perspective on their research topic?
- Do they talk about how their theoretical location shapes the way they analyze and interpret their results? They may also talk about how the act of conducting and analyzing their research altered the theoretical location they started from.
- In describing their personal, social and theoretical relationship with their research, researchers need to choose what elements to describe. Do you think what they describe helps you understand the role these elements played in their data collection and analysis?

Theoretical framework

Most qualitative research identifies the theoretical perspective that lies behind the research, although the authors may not always do so explicitly. Some theoretical perspectives are what we call 'macro' perspectives, that is, they address large domains about the way the world is and how people behave. You can understand the macro-perspective of a researcher by asking yourself:

- Are they studying how people **experience** something (e.g., a life event such as a birth or chronic illness)? In philosophy, this is called **phenomenology**, the study of the structure of experience.
- Are they studying how people come to **know** things (e.g., from family, education, media, society at large) or what they consider **knowledge** (e.g., that immunization is safe or not safe for children) or how health knowledge is socially created (e.g., by whether a community has a Western-style medical clinic or a healer practising traditional medicine)? In philosophy, this is called **epistemology**, the study of what constitutes knowledge and how we know it.
- Are they studying issues central to our **being** as humans such as our moral and ethical being, or our relationship with death? In philosophy, this is called **ontology**, the study of the nature of being, existence, or reality.

Within macro-level theories, there are many 'middle-range' theories that allow researchers to use the abstract concepts of macro-level theories to help design research on specific social and health issues. Here are some of the major ones you are likely to encounter in the QL health literature:

> **Positivism**: You may encounter discussion of positivism in QL research, but not as an approach that the researchers themselves are adopting. In the positivist approach, reality is seen as stable, fixed and measurable, and a 'right' explanation can be discovered for all phenomena if we search long and hard enough. This perspective lies at the heart of QN research, and is frequently criticized by QL researchers as inappropriate and not very useful for studying the complex, unpredictable behaviour of individuals and social groups.

> **Interpretative approaches**: In opposition to positivism, QL researchers prefer to speak of the way we interpret reality, rather than about an objective reality.

> **Social constructionism**: This approach sees reality as something that is socially constructed. For example, thanks in part to media, Western society equates thinness with health and moral goodness. It associates obesity, as measured by the BMI (Body Mass Index) with disease and moral failure. These theorists, however, would argue that 'obesity' is as much a social construction as it is a medical one, and that BMI, a measure originally developed within the insurance industry, is not only an inaccurate predictor of health status but it also has negative social and psychological consequences.

> **Critical theory approaches**: Critical theory approaches focus on power inequities within society that are based on gender, class, race, and other social constructs.

> **Feminist approaches**: Feminism, which was originally a movement devoted to gender issues and to achieving equality for women, has now expanded to consider intersecting issues that create power inequities. For example, although it is true globally that women experience inequity relative to men, the problems are worse for women of colour or women living in poverty or in developing countries that were previously colonized.

> **Participatory approaches**: This approach sees research as co-constructed by researchers and participants, on the basis that although researchers are experts in the sense of formal academic training, the participants are the experts of their own lives and communities.

All theories are based on 'assumptions', that is, a belief that is used as the basis of an idea. For example, in the theoretical approaches given above, critical theory assumes that there are unequal power relationships in any society while the participatory approach assumes that people will work together collaboratively to achieve a common benefit.

Research design and methods

Here are the broad QL research approaches commonly used in the nursing literature:

Phenomenological (note, phenomenology is both a philosophy and a research method): The purpose of this research is to capture the 'lived experience' of participants. Their experiences are collected from a small number of participants through observation, interviews, video and audiotapes, and descriptions written by the participants. The researcher then examines the captured materials and attempts to describe them by staying as close to the 'phenomena' (the experiences) as possible. Phenomenological philosophy is used to describe and interpret the meanings the researcher derives from the data. When you read phenomenological research, ask yourself:

- Does the researcher attempt to stay close to the personal meaning described by the participant?
- Is the participant's 'voice' reflected in the interpretation or description?

Ethnographic: The aim of ethnography is to learn and understand cultural phenomena, which reflect the knowledge and system of meanings within the life of a cultural group. Culture is defined in many ways, and as a term is sometimes applied very broadly, such as to an entire racialized group (sometimes offensively broad, as when people speak of 'Aboriginal' or 'Hispanic' culture, as though any statement about culture could be true when applied to so many individuals in and from so many places). Or the word can be applied as narrowly as to describe the group experience of nurses in a single labour/delivery unit. One type of ethnographic research is called **community-based participatory research**. This research is conducted as an equal partnership between the formally trained researcher and the members of a community. The community and researcher collaborate at every stage, from deciding what problem to investigate, defining it, deciding on a research design, gathering resources, carrying out the research, interpreting the results, sharing the credit, and deciding how to put the results into action in the community. Ask yourself if you see this. If not, does the researcher tell you why? Or do you feel the researcher had unequal power in directing the research – if so, in what ways?

Grounded theory: grounded theory is related to phenomenological research in that it studies phenomena; for example, the stress and burnout experienced by newly graduated nurses. The intent of grounded theory as it was originally developed by Glaser and Strauss (1967) is to develop a theory that explains the phenomenon being studied. The name refers to the idea that the theory is 'grounded' in the data from which it emerges. In grounded theory, the researcher collects, organizes and analyzes data, and forms theory all at the same time. Data are collected from multiple sources and constantly compared with each other in order to code and categorize them into themes from which the theory is developed. Currently, however, it is not unusual for researchers to conduct a form of grounded theory research without necessarily developing a theory.

Historical: It is only by understanding where we have come from that we can truly understand who we are. For this reason, there is an ever-growing body of nursing research concerned with the history of nursing as a profession and the history of nursing knowledge. Unlike other forms of QL research, the 'participants' may no longer be living, so these researchers rely on historical 'artefacts', that is, documents, photos, journals, legal documents, historical archives, newspapers, and other forms of primary documentation that survive from the period under study and help the researcher build a picture of the values, beliefs and knowledge of society as it was. For example, through the historical evidence we have about Florence Nightingale's life, we can come to understand that it was her upper-class status – in the rigid class structure of Victorian England – which allowed her to advocate on the highest levels of government for the nursing profession. That allows us to make a comparison with the power structures of our own times and the challenges faced by nursing and midwifery around the world.

Whatever approach is used, the design of a QL study needs to be 'feasible'. By this we mean, is it doable? It should be practically feasible: ask yourself if the researcher has the personal qualities, life history, and training to gain access to and 'fit in' with the lives of the people or organizational culture being explored. Another part of practical feasibility involves resources, both of time and materials (including funding). Access is another issue, especially in studying groups with high mobility, such as homeless adolescents. It is especially important for the design to be ethically feasible, because QL research is often conducted with vulnerable populations.

Sample and setting: Samples are often small and focused. Settings are usually 'natural', meaning that participants are studied where they live or work. Alternatively, the participant and researcher may arrange to meet in a 'neutral' setting that is convenient for the participant. Ask yourself these questions:

- What information is provided about the characteristics of the participants or organizational setting? Does that information help you understand the interaction with the researcher and the data that were produced as a result?
- What information is provided about how the researcher recruited the participants? Why these particular participants? Did any of them decline to participate and if so, why? Do the researchers explain how they addressed ethical concerns? Do they describe any important ethical challenges in conducting research on this particular group of participants – for example, studying women in relationships where they are the victims of domestic violence might create safety issues for them. Did the researchers receive ethics approval from their own institution and any other appropriate organizations? Do they describe the process of getting informed consent from their participants? Do they persuade

you that there were no risks to their participants from participating? Were there any benefits to their participants?

- Do you think the group of people or organizational setting is relevant to your own practice and patients? What do you feel you are learning from reading about them?

Generating and collecting data

- Do they describe how they generated or collected their data, and why they chose that method?
- If the researcher[s] modified the methods during the study (as frequently happens in qualitative research as part of the emergent design process), do they explain how this came about?
- Do they explain clearly what form the data were collected in (e.g., written documents such as surveys, researcher field notes, audio tapes, video)?
- How did they generate their data? Here are some common ways:
  - participant/non-participant observation
  - field notes
  - reflexive journals
  - interviews
  - focus groups and key informant interviews
  - analysis of documents and other materials
  - surveys and questionnaires

Interviews: Interviews, with individuals or with groups (e.g., focus groups) are the most common source of data for QL health researchers. They are categorized as structured, semi-structured or in-depth. In a structured interview, the questions are carefully scripted, with every participant being asked exactly the same questions in the same order. For a semi-structured interview, the researcher designs a guide that sets an agenda for the interview, but allows the interviewees to speak to each item as they choose. In an in-depth interview, questions are 'open-ended'. They are designed to act as topic openers for the participant to take in any direction they like, and subsequent questions are then based on what the interviewee offers. Interviews are a wonderful window into the inner world of participants, revealing what they think and feel about their lives and experiences. But interviews don't necessarily give a clear picture of how people behave, which may be very different from how they say in an interview that they behave.

Observational studies: Observational studies, as the name suggests, allow researchers to describe and understand what is going on in a particular social setting. They do not intervene to direct or control what happens, and the data they collect is the naturally occurring talk and behaviours of people's everyday lives and interactions.

Case studies: 'Case study' is a broad term, referring to the process of studying a phenomenon within its context (Green and Thorogood,

2004, p.36). Case studies are used in both QN and QL research, and in fact were used in QN long before QL came along. In QL, 'case' may be applied widely – for example, funding of a women's HIV/AIDS support program (the phenomenon) and its impact within its context, in this case a historically poor neighbourhood in the capital city of Namibia, a country with one of the world's highest HIV/AIDS rates.

At the other end of the spectrum, the case that is studied may be a single person – a 'life history'. An example would be collecting the life story of a person who has been in and out of mental institutions and jail since his teens. There is great value in learning such a story, as it illuminates the failures within the mental health and judicial systems.

Surveys and questionnaires: The basic idea of a survey or questionnaire is the same whether a study is quantitative or qualitative: it is a means of collecting the same set of data from every 'case' in the study (Green and Thorogood, 2004, p.36). In the case of QN research, however, the purpose is to narrowly control the responses so that the data collected can then be expressed in numeric form. A 'purely' qualitative survey, on the other hand, would use only open-ended questions. In actuality, a great many QL surveys and questionnaires use questions of both kinds, for example, collecting demographic data before offering a set of semi-structured or open-ended questions.

Data analysis

- Do they describe their findings clearly?
- Do they describe the process they went through to analyze their findings?
- Do they explain how they chose which data to analyze, and what they chose to omit?
- If they used a grounded theory approach, do they explain how they derived their categories/themes from their data? Does it seem to you that the themes that emerged in their analysis are reflected in their examples and quotations? Grounded theory methods that seek patterns (such as coding, concept mapping, emerging themes) should leave you with a feeling of rich description. They should also leave you with a clear sense of how the theoretical concepts the researcher began from have contributed to the analysis.
- How do they interpret their findings?
- If relevant, do they try to establish the following elements of their analysis? Remember, these concepts may not be relevant to all QL studies:
  - Rigour: the pursuit at all stages of a study of accuracy and precision.
  - Transferability: the extent to which the results can be transferred to a larger population. In QN research, this is called 'generalizability'

and is established through statistical analysis. In QL, transferability is established by considering the kinds of relationships between the study sample and the larger group it represents.

- o Credibility: this is not an easy dimension to appraise, though its dictionary meaning is fairly straightforward: 'the quality of deserving to be believed and trusted' (LDCE). Those who are experienced in conducting and reading QL research are able to draw on their knowledge of previous studies; they also have background knowledge about the historical/social/political/theoretical contexts of the research. Nonetheless, students who are still learning these dimensions can ask themselves: 'Based on my appraisal of everything I've read in this study and about the researcher, do I feel convinced?'
- o Other terms you may encounter are 'dependability', 'confirmability', 'coherence', and 'authenticity'.

The narrative of a QL representation

We said above the QL is language-based, so you need to carefully consider the narrative of a study, that is, the story it tells. You also need to distinguish between the participant's narrative and the researcher's narrative. The former is that of the interviews; the latter is that of the researcher's interpretation or representation. The narrative dimension is especially relevant to ethnographic studies because they attempt to portray the concepts of physical and social health/illness in terms of people's lived experience:

- Is the writing richly detailed in describing both the facts about the participants and their feelings? Do you feel immersed in their lives?
- Is there a sense of the past and future of the participants, not just their present situation? Do you feel you are sharing in their life's journey?
- Does it touch you on an emotional level? Do you perhaps feel a connection between their lives and yours, or does the contrast help you understand your own life and practice in a new way?
- Is it an ethical narrative? That is, do you feel that there is mutual respect and sensitivity between the researcher[s] and participants?
- Does the narrative satisfy you rationally, so you feel convinced that the results mean what the authors say they do?

Conclusion: how valuable is the research?

- Do they consider how their research may be used? Do they discuss the contribution their study makes? It may be a contribution to the body of current research on the topic. It may contribute to practice, policy or social and community action. It may contribute to our understanding of health within the context of social life.
- Do they identify new areas for research, or ways to continue their current research?

FOR FURTHER READING

Burns, N. and Grove, S.K. (1995) *Understanding Nursing Research*. Philadelphia, PA: W.B. Saunders.

Creswell, J.W. (2003) *Research Design: Qualitative, quantitative, and mixed method approaches.* Thousand Oaks, CA: Sage Publications.

Critical Skills Appraisal Programme (CASP). Making sense of evidence: CASP critical appraisal checklist for qualitative studies. Available at www.casp-uk. net/

Denzin, N.K. and Lincoln, Y.S. (2011) *The SAGE Handbook of Qualitative Research* (4th edn). Thousand Oaks, CA: Sage Publications.

Domholdt, E.A. (1993) *Physical Therapy Research: Principles and applications.* Philadelphia, PA: W.B. Saunders.

Eakin, J.M. and Mykhalovskiy, E. (2003) 'Reframing the evaluation of qualitative health research', *Journal of Evaluation in Clinical Practice*, 9(2): 187–94.

Glaser, B.G. and Strauss, A.L. (1967) *The Discovery of Grounded Theory: Strategies for qualitative research.* Chicago, IL: Aldine.

Goubil-Gambrell, P. (1992) *A Practitioner's Guide to Research Methods.* Technical communication.

Green, J. and Thorogood, N. (2004) *Qualitative Methods for Health Research.* London: Sage.

Neutens, J. and Robinson, L. (2001) *Research Techniques for the Health Sciences* (3rd edn). Toronto, ON: Benjamin Cummings.

WRITING UP YOUR LITERATURE REVIEW

> **OVERVIEW**
>
> - Introducing the review
> - The body of the review
>   - Structuring the body
>   - Learning to 'speak citation': the discourse of citations
>   - Verbs and their persuasive power
>   - The importance of qualifying
>   - Describing the evidence
> - Concluding the review

Traditionally, the literature review occupies the second chapter of the thesis, providing a rationale for the research objectives or questions that follow (or in some cases precede). In many cases, there are two literature review chapters, one to review the research literature and one for the theoretical literature. This is especially common when the research work is qualitative. Discussion of the literature returns in later chapters, when the ways in which the study's results support, contrast, and/or add to the existing literature are argued. The ultimate goals of the review chapter[s] are to leave the reader persuaded that: a) there is previous research/theory that supports conducting your research; and b) there is a gap in the literature that your research is going to help fill.

All of the writing strategies and language suggestions in this chapter are intended to help you convince the examiners of the following:

1. You have developed comprehensive search skills, have a solid knowledge base of the literature, and keep current with it – you have established your credentials as a researcher.
2. You are able to frame your own work as belonging to the scholarly group you and your examiners are part of – you have authority as a member of your scholarly community.

3. If there is anything relevant that will be omitted in your own study, it is because others have already sufficiently dealt with it.
4. There is a gap in our knowledge that your research can fill.

INTRODUCING THE REVIEW

It is very common to include a brief overview paragraph at the beginning of each chapter, giving a broad overview of the chapter and its purpose, such as this one from JL:

> In this chapter, I provide a critical review of the literature. The purpose of this review is to explore current constructions of and knowledge about patients' experiences of the technological in heart surgery. Specific attention was directed at the components of patients' experiential accounts.

Next, the introduction describes how you conducted your comprehensive search for all the relevant literature. The goal is to persuade the reader that you looked everywhere you should have, looked for the right things, excluded the irrelevant, and ended with a sufficiently large and comprehensive body of literature to review. In searching for the literature, you may have encountered one of two ends of a spectrum. If you found very little previous research, you need to explain why there has been so little, in other words, that the lack of research is not because the topic isn't really worth pursuing. You also have to explain what you did to expand your search to include other, related literatures that add depth to your review. On the other hand, when there is a very great deal of previous research, you need to argue that the topic is not yet 'mined out' and that you are able to make that all-important original contribution.

It is common to provide an outline of the search strategy you used to identify and retrieve the research. If you are doing this, include a description of the criteria you used to select the reports included in the review (e.g., the problem, the population and the setting, and the type of research methods, or whatever your criteria were). Identify the total number of studies that your search revealed and the final number meeting your criteria.

It is important not just to say what literature you included (and why) but also what you excluded (and why), as KE does:

> The research studies that used the constructs of leadership, medication errors, absenteeism, intent to leave, job satisfaction and quality of care were assessed using the Cooper (1982) guidelines ... . Research articles that were not peer reviewed were excluded. The research studies that described or compared leadership programs were excluded because they were outside the topic of the proposed study. Research articles that did not describe the methodology, provide the instruments used, or address the reliability and validity of the instruments were excluded. The literature review is organized into the general areas of study for this research study: leadership, nurse, patient and system outcomes. (KE, p.14)

An improvement in terms of writing style would be to avoid so many repetitions of 'were excluded', in this way, for example:

> Research articles were excluded if they met the following criteria: 1) were not peer-reviewed; 2) described or compared leadership programmes, because they were outside

the topic of the proposed study; or 3) did not describe the methodology, provide the instruments used, or address the reliability and validity of the instruments.

JL faced a complicating factor in conducting her review because little research dealt explicitly with her topic. This is not an uncommon problem – after all, you are trying to make an original contribution and may be striking out in areas others have not yet explored. As a result, JL needed to broaden the scope of her review and now she has to justify that choice. She begins with her overview statement about the topic of the review, but very soon raises the issue (in italics):

> At the outset of this review, I found an absence of empirical literature that focused specifically on patients' experiences of the technological in heart surgery. Nevertheless, the technological emerged implicitly in researchers' analytic summaries and participants' narratives in the studies reviewed. This implicitness may be a result of the prevalence of the technological in everyday life – it is so present that it is viewed as ordinary and mundane. *Considering the implicit nature of the technological in the literature it was necessary to broaden the scope of the review to research concerning patients' experiences of heart surgery more broadly. This was a critical portal* to understanding how patients narrate the technological in heart surgery and how identity and moral issues are framed in these accounts. (p.27; italics added)

In the final part of the introduction, give the reader a clear description of the organization of the chapter. In this example, the connectors that draw MRV's reader through his outline are italicized. He signals the purpose of the paragraph with 'In this chapter':

> In this chapter, the *initial sections* explain immigration patterns and socio-demographic structures of South Asian emigrants in the UK. The *subsequent sections* introduce South Asians' perspectives on health and illness, cultural and religious beliefs and practices around end of life. *Further sections* explore the views and experiences of health professionals involved in caring for South Asians with palliative care needs. This chapter *concludes* by summarising the gaps identified in current knowledge and lists out the aim and objects of this research study.

THE BODY OF THE REVIEW

Structuring the body

The point of a review is not merely to string together separate appraisals of individual studies, so it is not enough to go through the sources one by one and just summarize them. The objective is to pull together a coherent argument that your research study is supported by strong evidence. To do this, the literature must be analyzed (broken down into its constituent parts) and then synthesized (brought together to demonstrate its overall strengths and limits).

A chapter-length review should be divided into sub-sections. Each sub-section might begin with a few paragraphs that summarize the common strengths, weaknesses, methodologies or findings shared by a relatively large group of studies. Following that, the most important and relevant studies can be focused on individually and/or in comparison to each other. The important and most relevant studies can be described in detail. It is important to provide comparable information for each one (e.g., participants and setting, variables, design, results/conclusions), advancing an argument about its strengths/weaknesses and relationship with your research study. The sub-section ends with a brief summary.

Your breakdown of the literature (analysis) and bringing it together (synthesis) in a way that paves the way for your study should highlight unanswered questions and methodological problems with past studies. By the end, the rationale for what you propose (your questions) and why you propose to carry out your research a certain way (your methodology) should be obvious.

Green and Macauley (2007) found that some of the doctoral students they interviewed adopted mind-mapping and other meta-cognition strategies to find and organize the literature. As one student said,

> I actually approach [information seeking and organization] from a mind-mapping approach, where I identify around a half dozen subtopics both from experience and from my early dips into the literature … starting some database inquiries and seeing what I come up with. And in the beginning you're trying to find out what terms other people have used. … And then I get my subtopics and I inquire around those and I look for overlaps. (p.324)

There are a variety of ways to organize the sub-sections, such as the following:

> *Chronologically:* This is useful when tracing the development of, for example, theoretical frameworks, history of the profession or research methodologies (e.g., tools, instruments, interventions), or how we came to the state of current knowledge. In this passage introducing a sub-section in her review, FWM outlines the history of an area where our knowledge is still very limited. The wording that traces her argument about the research efforts is italicized. The first sentence identifies the unresolved issue:

The extent to which the two branches of the autonomic nervous system play a role in hypertensive pregnancy is not clear. *Early research* of sympathetic nervous system activity in pre-eclampsia, *using indirect measures* such as catecholamine levels and hemodynamic changes, *found conflicting results. It has since been demonstrated, with more rigorous research designs and direct microelectrode measures* of sympathetic nerve output, that women with pregnancy hypertension have … . (FWM, pp.8–9)

> *By themes:* Here, JL uses the simple, effective device of a numbered list to identify her sub-sections:

This synthesis is organized according to themes that inductively emerged from the literature, following a thematic analysis. I critically examine and synthesize the six thematic areas that emerged: (1) body; (2) mortality; (3) psychological dimensions; (4) spirituality; (5) activities of daily living (ADL), roles and relationships; and (6) quality of life (QOL) and functionality. (JL, p.27)

> *By populations:*

In this chapter, *the initial sections* explain immigration patterns and socio-demographic structures of *South Asian emigrants in the UK.* The subsequent *sections* introduce *South Asians'* perspectives on health and illness, cultural and religious beliefs and practices around end of life. *Further sections* explore the views and experiences of *health professionals* involved in caring for South Asians with palliative care needs. (MRV, pp.23–4)

> *By outcomes:*

The literature review is organized into the general areas of study for this research study: *leadership, nurse, patient and system outcomes.* (KE, p.14)

> *By related independent and dependent variables:*

The following literature review has been organized into three general categories:

physiology of blood pressure control; hypertension in pregnancy; and mind-body communication and psychophysiologic therapies, under which guided imagery as clinical intervention for blood pressure and anxiety is specifically addressed. (FWM, p.6)

> *By research design and methodology:* Begin with weaker designs (bearing in mind that they may also have something to contribute to your study) and progress to stronger ones. You would choose this option if it is especially important to justify your own choice of study design. In this case, the final design you discuss is the one you wish to use, in other words, the design that is strongest for what you need to accomplish. In assessing methodological issues, also consider what conclusions they come to: are they somewhat similar despite the methodological problems?

> *By theoretical premises:* As mentioned above, if your study is qualitative or mixed-methods, it is likely that you will devote an entire chapter to reviewing the theoretical literature. Such an organization might cover definitions, conceptualizations and ways to operationalize a concept such as, for example, 'culture' or 'complexity'.

SOURCE

Green, R. and Macauley, P. (2007) 'Doctoral students' engagement with information: An American-Australian perspective'. *Libraries and the Academy* 7(3), 317–32.

Learning to 'speak citation': the discourse of citations

Learning to 'speak citation' is a requirement for becoming a full member of the research community. In the process of writing a literature review, you learn what, when, how, and how much to cite, as well as the rhetorical function of verbs and modifiers that describe and evaluate the works cited.

In the process of searching the literature, tracking citations among articles is an extremely efficient way of learning the scope of research on a topic across time, methodologies and results. Tracking citations not only helps in developing this understanding of the field, it also makes clear the spheres of influence within it. These processes of understanding, quietly developing as the search is conducted, come to fruition in the thinking process of writing the literature review. The way you use and refer to citations in writing up the review demonstrates your understanding of the spheres of influence and your position within – or contrary to – those spheres.

Phrases that signal consensus:

As is well known …

Some/many/most authors/scholars/researchers agree that …

It is widely accepted that …

A widely held belief/idea/notion is …

It has been widely reported that …

The scholarly consensus is/seems to be that …

A large/substantial body of research has consistently demonstrated that …

The most widely accepted explanation is …

A common theoretical position is …

Most authors would interpret this as …

This is generally interpreted as …

Our present understanding of … is …

A widespread practice is to …

It has been shown repeatedly that …

Phrases that signal contrasting work:

Another view is that …

A competing theory …

In contrast, …

Phrases that indicate quantity:

A wealth of literature

Many noteworthy studies

A great many explanations have been advanced

Several explanations have been proposed for …

Some authors have suggested that …

Several authors have commented on …

A large/small number of studies

Many/some/only a few studies

A large/small body of research

Researchers have only recently turned to …

… has been the focus of numerous/various/some studies …

Phrases that show the development of our knowledge over time:

Originally suggested by …

Early research proposed that …

Research conducted in the 19xxs paved the way for …

A long history of research

Cornerstone

Groundwork

Of fundamental importance was the discovery by … that …

This idea derives from …

In a preliminary study, [Name] showed …

Exploratory work was carried out by … who demonstrated that …

[Name] first put forward the idea that …

[Name]'s initial development of …

Our understanding was further developed by

X marked a major turning point in …

[Name]'s work had a profound influence on …

[Name]'s study is a classic example of …

Previous studies of … have shown/suggested that …

Results from earlier studies indicated that …

X was linked to Y in studies that …

This led some authors to suggest that …

… also contributed to the development of …

Until recently, …

It was previously believed that … but we now know that …

An area that has become increasingly important

The conventional understanding of … is/was

Based on these results, …

Historically

Traditionally

Showing relationship:

The current study is based in part on …

My work builds on …

The X tool was adapted for this study

A number of other studies also focus on …

… complements existing research

Similar/contrasting results have been found in …

This interpretation is supported by earlier work on …

This supports the view that …

Another view is that …

This is reflected in [Name]'s findings that …

Other authors have also called for …

Researchers adopting this position include …

Verbs and their persuasive power

We use verbs to indicate strength or weakness. We also use neutral verbs for the purpose of description.

To indicate a study makes a strong case for its results:

shows

demonstrates

establishes

Note: adding 'conclusively' or 'strongly' or 'convincingly' to any of the above increases the sense of strength.

makes a valuable contribution to …

a valuable and important study of …

an important and original work

a comprehensive examination of …

an in-depth discussion of …

The results lend strong support to …

suggest a number of new avenues for research

To indicate a study's conclusions can be accepted for now but that more research is needed:

suggest

indicate

attempt (can also be used as a negative: 'Study X attempted to establish but ultimately failed')

To describe neutrally:

Their results reveal

They found that

Findings revealed

analyze

carry out

conduct

describe

develop

discuss

do

expand

explain

explore

find

focus

illustrate

note

observe

point out

present

remark

replicate

say

state

study

To describe the argument a study makes:

These verbs work well with sentence structures such as 'The authors [verb] that …' or 'The study [verb] that …':

advocates

argues

concludes

emphasizes

holds the position that

maintains

makes the case that

proposes

suggests

attempts to show

To indicate serious limitations:

The study lacks …

While it may be the case that … , this study

The author's claim is not well founded

The extent to which this reflects … is unclear

The authors overlook

[Names] present no new insights into …

were strongly biased

failed to establish

omitted to …

does not account for

has failed to gain acceptance

does not adequately demonstrate

Critics would argue that …

[Names] give a detailed but flawed analysis of …

Signalling debate:

One of the issues currently under discussion

foremost in current debates

Another view is that

has been hotly debated

This study questions the widely held view that …

Words and phrases that signal current influence:

noteworthy

important (*the most commonly used; beware of overusing it*) significant (*be careful to qualify this word if you are not using it in the sense of statistical significance. For example, politically significant, a significant development, significant to the community, etc.*)

influential work

The most detailed examination to date …

an important advance

The last few years have witnessed a shift from … to …

a recent surge of interest in …

a comparatively recent focus

has attracted considerable intention

an increasing amount of literature

promising new avenue

a new way of looking at

the well-established principle that …

Signalling the need for more research:

A number of aspects require further investigation

Further study is needed to determine …

Very little is known about …

No clear evidence exists that …

Little attention has been given to …

There has been no systematic examination of …

… is not yet clearly understood

The question remains, however,

Although much has been learned in recent years, a number of questions remain.

While the initial findings are promising, more research is required to …

The importance of qualifying

This has nothing to do with the Tour de France. To 'qualify' means to add words or phrases to something being said, in order to limit or add to its meaning. Qualification is an important tool, because research design and writing resist certainty – it's why we so rarely see the word 'prove' unless it relates to mathematical proof. The purpose of research is to ask and answer questions, not to establish absolute truth. For this reason, we make subtle distinctions in our writing around how closely we come to 'proof' or 'truth'. Compare these, for example:

- Most scholars agree that …
- Most scholars would agree that …

Neither claims that everyone agrees, but the first indicates that there is currently a general state of agreement within the literature. The second is less certain – if scholars had the opportunity, they would surely agree but haven't actually done so. The next level down would be

- Many scholars agree that …

Further qualification downward, such as

- Many scholars would agree that …

weakens the claim of agreement still more, suggesting that in fact the majority of scholars do *not* agree.

Common qualifiers include:

Would, could, should, might, may, can

It is probable/likely that

It is possible that

Many, most

Some, a few, only a few

Although

FOR FURTHER READING

Howe, S. and Henriksson, K. (2002) *Phrase Book for Writing Papers and Research*. Cambridge, UK: Whole World Company Press.

Describing the evidence

All argument must be supported with evidence, so a major component of a review is description – of history, demographics, social issues, research studies, and other types of evidence we use to support our arguments.

Description ultimately has an argumentative function, but in academic writing it adopts a neutral tone. This tone can be a challenge for writers who feel passionately about, for example, a social or political issue around healthcare. Unfortunately, a tone that reflects the emotions of the writer makes the reader feel she or he is biased. A neutral description, therefore, is always more persuasive. The intent of the description is simply to provide evidence to support an argumentative claim. For example, in this paragraph of his review, MRV presents statistics to support his claim that based on the ethnic demographic structure of the UK, South Asians are an important population to study:

According to the Office of National Statistics (ONS) Census 2001, nearly 7.9 % of the population in the UK is made up of people from ethnic minority groups. In the 2001 census, South Asian populations had grown 53% compared to 1991, due to factors such as a high birth rate and net international immigration among these populations (Hatton 2005). South Asians constitute the single largest ethnic minority group (50.3% of ethnic population) in the United Kingdom; in particular, Indians and Pakistanis respectively made up 1.8% and 1.3% of the total population of the UK in the ONS Census 2001. In some cities such as Bradford, London, and Leeds, South Asians make up the majority of the inner city population, exceeding the majority (CRE 2005, 2007). Table 1 explains the population of the UK by ethnic group, based on the ONS 2001 Census. (MRV, p.26)

CONCLUDING THE REVIEW

The conclusion of the review usually has two sub-sections:

1. a summary of what you have presented in the chapter, and a concluding statement that ties the support/gaps in the literature to the purpose (and theoretical framework where applicable) of your research;
2. a statement of your research objectives/questions/hypotheses.

1. The concluding statement:

KE's summary is an excellent example of a brief paragraph that clearly places her own research as part of the literature and advancing it:

Summary

[1] There is empirical evidence suggesting a relationship between leadership and staff retention and positive patient outcomes. [2] Prior research has identified the need for further studies regarding the linkage between leadership practices and nurse, patient and system outcomes. [3] The literature reviewed provides support for the selection of variables for this study. [4] The current study adds to the nursing leadership research and literature by examining hospital nurse managers' use of leadership practices and exploring the relationship between nurse, patient and system outcomes. [5] Specifically this study examined the nurse outcomes of absenteeism and intent to leave, the patient outcome as the medication errors, and the system outcome as the staff nurses' perception of the quality of patient care and nursing care on the hospital unit. (KE, p.40)

[1] states the conclusion of the review, i.e., that it produced empirical evidence to support undertaking a study of her research problem.

[2] more specific detail links the gap she identified with her own research objectives.

[3] demonstrates that her study variables derive from previous research.

[4] positions her study within the scholarly community by identifying the contribution it will make to the literature.

[5] gives specifics of the study's contribution to the literature but also provides a transition to the upcoming description of the study design in the Methods chapter.

2. Stating the research questions

In a published study, the research objectives and questions are given at the end of the literature review, and this is true of most dissertations as well. The other possible positions are at the end of the Introduction chapter or the beginning of the Methods chapter. Unless your supervisor suggests one of these, however, the literature review chapter is the default position.

To understand how to write this section, it's important to distinguish among research purposes, goals, aims, objectives, questions and hypotheses.

The **research purpose, goal or aim** follows from your development of the problem in the Introduction chapter. A purpose, goal or aim identifies and describes the change to the problem the researchers hope will result from their study. For example, in a study of the problem of inadequate nutrient intake among pregnant women, the change the researchers hope for is evidence that dietary supplements might alleviate the problem, and the aim might be the following:

> To evaluate the nutrient intake of Finnish pregnant women and relate it to the use of vitamin/mineral supplements.

A **research objective** is more specific: it identifies and describes the independent and dependent variables that will be studied to address the problem. For example, an objective might be:

> To measure nutrient intake adequacy of vitamin/mineral supplement users and non-users among Finnish pregnant women.

Notice that the language here signals that the study design is a randomized controlled trial because it contains all the PICO components: population (pregnant women), intervention (supplements), comparison (users and non-users) and outcome (nutrient intake adequacy).

More specific still, a **research question** is an interrogative statement that the researchers develop to direct their study. For example:

> What is the nutrient intake adequacy of Finnish pregnant women who use vitamin/mineral supplements compared to non-users?

KE's research questions are stated at the end of her Introduction chapter and they follow from her statement of purpose. The key aspect to note here is how precisely the questions are worded. Also, all key words and phrases are repeated each time because each question must stand alone. Finally, they use identical ('parallel') structures that make it easy for the reader to see how they are the same and where they differ. I have used ellipsis (…) to indicate the list of five leadership practices that are the same in each question.

Purpose of the study

[1] The purpose of the study was twofold: (1) to describe the nurse managers' leadership practices as perceived by staff nurses, and (2) to examine the relationship between the staff nurses' perceptions of the nurse managers' leadership practices and the following outcomes: staff absenteeism, staff intent to leave, medication errors, and the

staff perception of the quality of patient care and the quality of nursing care. [2] Using Kouzes and Posner's theory of leadership (2001), this study examined the relationships between the five leadership practices: Challenge the process, Inspire a shared vision, Enable others to act, Model the way, and Encourage the heart and the selected staff and patient outcomes in a Saskatchewan hospital environment. (KE, p.7)

[1] describes the twofold purpose, clearly delineated with numbers.

[2] links the research questions to her theoretical framework.

Research questions

1. What are the staff nurses' perceptions of the nurse managers' use of the leadership practices: Challenge the process, Inspire a shared vision, Enable others to act, Model the way, and Encourage the heart? [answers the first purpose to describe practices]
2. What is the relationship between staff nurses' perceptions of nurse manager leadership practices (…) and staff absenteeism? [each subsequent question addresses one of the outcomes being studied in the same order they were listed in the Purpose paragraph]
3. What is the relationship between staff nurses' perceptions of nurse manager leadership practices (…) and staff intent to leave?
4. What is the relationship between staff nurses' perceptions of nurse manager leadership practices (…) and medication errors?
5. What is the relationship between staff nurses' perception of nurse manager leadership practices (…) and the staff perception of quality of patient care and nursing care on the unit? (KE, pp.7–8)

Question 1 addresses the first part of the purpose; each of questions 2–5 addresses one of the outcomes mentioned in the second part of the purpose, in exactly the same order.

Finally, a **hypothesis** is 'the formal statement of the expected relationship(s) between two or more variables in a specified population' (Burns and Grove, 1995, p.116). Hypotheses must be testable, that is, supported by statistical analysis of the data collected. As Burns and Grove explain, studies might have one or multiple hypotheses depending on the complexity of the study. They can belong to one of four categories:

(1) associative versus causal: if one changes, the other changes, in a positive or negative direction (Terms such as 'more' or 'less', 'increase' or 'decrease', 'higher' or 'lower' indicate the direction of the relationship),

(2) simple (i.e., two variables) versus complex (i.e., three or more variables),

(3) directional (i.e., associative or causal) versus nondirectional (i.e., a relationship exists but it is unclear whether the change occurs in positive or negative direction)

(4) null versus research: a research hypothesis states that there is a relationship between two or more variables; a null hypothesis states the same hypothesis but as a negative statement (e.g., 'There is no relationship …' or 'There is no difference …'). Null hypotheses are used for statistical testing and interpreting statistical outcomes. (Burns and Grove, 1995, p.117)

For example, a testable, associative (positive), simple research hypothesis would be:

Nutrient intake adequacy will be improved in Finnish pregnant women who use vitamin/mineral supplements compared to non-users.

SOURCES

Burns, N. and Grove, S.K. (1995) *Understanding Nursing Research*. Philadelphia, PA: W.B. Saunders.

Green, R. and Macauley, P. (2007) 'Doctoral students' engagement with information: An American-Australian perspective', *Libraries and the Academy*, 7(3): 317–32.

Howe, S. and Henriksson, K. (2002) *Phrase Book for Writing Papers and Research*. Cambridge, UK: Whole World Company Press.

9

WRITING UP THE METHODS, RESULTS AND FINAL CHAPTERS

OVERVIEW

- Methods in quantitative research
- Methodology and analysis in qualitative research
- Writing up the results of quantitative research
- Tables and figures
- Writing up the results of qualitative research: developing a voice
- Discussion: positioning yourself in the field
- Combining results with discussion
- The special case of the publication thesis
- Conclusions and other final bits

METHODS IN QUANTITATIVE RESEARCH

Nowhere is the narrative nature of a thesis more evident than in the Methods or Methodology chapter, which tells the story of your research in chronological order. In essence, this chapter describes what you did (your study design), in what order, how you did it, and why you did it that way. The goal is to tell the story so completely, accurately and precisely that another researcher could replicate your methods in future research and obtain the same results. The story has two parts: a) a full process description of your treatment/intervention procedure[s]; and b) a description of your measurements, including any statistical analyses.

A generic set of sections within the Methods chapter of a quantitative study would include these headings:

Participants

Inclusion criteria

Exclusion criteria

Study design

Interventions

Methods of measurement

Calculations

Analysis of data (Zeiger, 2000, p.135)

SOURCE

Zeiger, M. (2000) *Essentials of Writing Biomedical Research Papers* (2nd edn). New York: McGraw-Hill.

Here, however, we follow the story as it is structured in KE's methodology chapter. The purpose of KE's descriptive correlational study was 'to explore the relationship between nurse managers' leadership practices as measured by Kouzes and Posner's (2001) Leadership Practice Inventory and staff nurses' intent to leave the job, absenteeism, medication errors and the quality of care' (p.ii). She begins the chapter with an overview sentence of the kind we have been recommending, and her first heading ('Research design') follows immediately:

> This chapter describes the research design, setting, sample, instruments, and the procedure for data collection utilized in this research study. (KE, p.41)

Research design

KE's first step is to identify (italicized) and justify (bolded) the chosen design:

> *A non experimental, descriptive, correlational design using a survey method was utilized* for this study. This type of design **was chosen because** the researcher is interested in exploring the relationship between the leadership practices of nurse managers and selected nurse, patient and system outcomes. *A descriptive design was used* to describe the leadership practices of nurse managers as rated by their nursing staff using Kouzes and Posner's Leadership Practice Inventory (2002a). In a correlational design the researcher 'is **interested in quantifying the strength** of the relationship between the variables' (LoBiondo-Wood and Haber, 2006, p.242). A correlational design was used to examine the relationship between the leadership practices reported and specific outcomes including: … . The individual nurse was the unit of analysis for this research. (KE, p.41)

Note the significant use of passive verbs: *was utilized, was chosen, was used*. A passive verb has two related functions: it places the design of the study in the emphatic position at the start of the sentence or paragraph; it de-emphasizes the person doing the research in favour of the research itself. Passive verb constructions tend to figure prominently in Methods chapters.

Description of the setting

KE now describes her setting, beginning broadly (the city) and narrowing to the specific:

> The study was conducted in Regina, Saskatchewan, with the nursing staff from the two urban acute care hospitals in the Regina Qu'Appelle Health Region (RQHR). Regina,

the capital of Saskatchewan, is a city with a population of approximately 190,000. The only two acute care hospitals in the city serve as the referral centers for the southern half of Saskatchewan, a population of approximately 550,000. (KE, pp.41–2)

This brief description also justifies the choice of the setting – it serves a large, geographically diverse population in a major urban centre. From here, the next step is to describe the particular aspects of the setting that are relevant to the research. In KE's case, these are the size and type of units and the manager span of control (i.e., how many staff nurses report to a unit manager).

Sample

Describing the sample next is logical from the perspective of moving from broad to specific, as the sample exists within the setting. Obviously, it isn't enough simply to state the sample size and how it was arrived at – KE leads through the steps with a rationale provided for each one. I have left out her references and the actual calculations:

[1] The minimum sample sizes for correlational studies can be determined by using a formula (Israel, 1992) or estimated using a table (Yamane, 1967). [2] The sample size for this study was calculated using the formula … and then compared to the table [to arrive at] n = 308. This sample size of 308 participants is comparable to that estimated in the table (Appendix B) by Yamane (1967). [3] This sample size reflects the minimum number of obtained responses needed and not necessarily the number of surveys mailed. The average response rate for surveys mailed to the nursing population has been estimated at 35% (O'Brien-Pallas et al., 2005). [4] To maximize the percentage of obtained surveys, a total of 1000 nursing staff were randomly selected (the human resource department used a random number table) from the population of RNs and all of the LPNs at the two sites and mailed a package. [5] Since Site A has approximately double the number of nursing staff as Site B, the sample reflected the distribution by randomly selecting 700 staff from Site A and 300 staff from Site B. (KE, p.45)

[1] the two possible ways of arriving at the sample size.

[2] the next two sentences show how both were used.

[3] the rest of the paragraph details how many surveys were sent, using a randomized selection process, to obtain the desired responses.

[4] this is a very useful sentence structure: it begins with a short phrase to tell the reader why 1000 staff were selected.

[5] explains the distribution of selection using a similar grammatical structure, a clause (Since …) to begin the sentence.

Variables and measures

This is an extremely important section, because it lays the foundation for everything that follows. There can be no confidence in the study as a whole if the reader is not confident about the strength of its foundation, so this section both identifies the variables and measures, and argues for using them. In KE's case, she has five independent variables (leadership practices) derived from previous research by Kouzes and Posner and operationalized by the 30 questions of their Leadership Practices Inventory. She also has four dependent variables and a number of demographic characteristics. This complexity makes it an appropriate situation in which to use tables. Tables give the reader a clear overview of all this information, a reference as the reader goes through the measures that are systematically discussed in subsequent paragraphs. For each measure, description is combined with argument, as in these examples. In the first example, also note that the reader is referred to relevant appendix material in the first sentence.

Measure of leadership

Leadership Practice Inventory

The five leadership practices as described by Kouzes and Posner are the independent variables and are measured with the Leadership Practice Inventory (LPI, Appendix C). Written permission to use the LPI was obtained from Kouzes and Posner International (Appendix D). [description of LPI, its administration and scoring]. In their review of 18 leadership measurement tools, Huber et al. (2000) ranked Kouzes and Posner's LPI highest for psychometric properties and ease of use. (KE, p.48)

This is followed by sub-sections arguing for the reliability and validity of the LPI. Where there is strong support for reliability and validity, this is stated. Where there are potential problems, they are accounted for.

Measures of the outcomes

In this section, KE describes the measures of her outcomes and argues for their reliability and validity. Each sub-section is structured the same way: '*Name of outcome* – was measured by …' The following example demonstrates a way of stating the research support for the reliability and validity of a measure. The first sentence describes the measure (two questions); the second provides evidence of substantial research use of the measure; the third addresses a potential problem by citing that evidence; and the final sentence closes the argument with a logical connector ('Thus').

[1] *Staff nurse perceptions of Quality of Care* – was measured by asking respondents two questions: in the last year has the quality of patient care in the unit improved, remained the same or deteriorated, and would they describe the quality of nursing care during the last shift as excellent, good, fair or poor. [2] [describes the use of both questions in five previous studies, with sample sizes of 3016 to 10,184] [3] There are no documented psychometric tests for the two quality of care questions used in the current study; however, the questions have been used in five major studies nationally and internationally. [4] Thus, the questions used for the current study are the staff nurses' perception of the quality of patient care and nursing care. (KE, pp.58–9)

Data collection

In this section, KE not only describes the data collection process, she also introduces the important data collection documents included in her appendices. You'll notice that they are not mentioned in alphabetical order, apparently contrary to the rule that appendices are lettered in the order in which they appear in the text. However, KE has already mentioned these appendices and originally did so in order:

A stratified random sample was used for this study. The sample was stratified by hospital sites to reflect the population at the two sites: Site A has 906 staff nurses in the units eligible for this study and Site B has 439 staff nurses. A list of all eligible RNs and LPNs at the two hospital sites was generated by the RQHR human resource department, and a random list of 1000 names was obtained (using a random number table). There were 700 from Site A and 300 from Site B to keep the sample similar to the proportion of staff nurses at the two sites. After obtaining approval from the University of Toronto Ethics Board (Appendix I) and the RQHR Research Ethics Board (Appendix J) a three step mail out procedure was implemented (Brennan, 1992). A letter introducing the researcher and the study was mailed (Appendix E), then two weeks later an information letter (Appendix F) with the survey (Appendix G), containing the LPI questionnaire (Appendix C), and a self addressed postage paid return envelope was sent. The third step was a reminder letter (Appendix H) sent two weeks following the survey mailout. (KE, p.55)

Data analysis

This section needs to:

- identify and justify the statistical tests you used. In this example, note the shift in verb tense from past (what was done in the study) to present (describing what the tests do and why they are appropriate for this study)

Data on all variables **were summarized** using descriptive statistics. The relationship between each of the five [independent variables] and [four dependent variables] **was analyzed** using Pearson product-moment correlation coefficient (r), logistic and multiple regression analysis. **Pearson product-moment correlation coefficient is** a parametric test that **measures** the direction and strength of a linear relationship of two variables to describe the relationship (Green and Salkind, 2005). **Logistic regression is** a type of regression that **is used** when the dependent variables are dichotomous (Munro, 2005). **Multiple regression analysis is** the appropriate type of analysis for this correlational study because it **examines** the relationship between a continuous dependent variable and several independent variables (LoBiondo-Wood and Haber, 2006). (KE, pp.56–7)

- explain potential problems in the analysis and how they were resolved:

Some of the nurse managers could be identified by their unit as there is only one neurosciences, palliative, and neonatal unit. To address this potential the units were combined and numbered 1 through 10. (KE, p.57)

- explain discrepancies:

One explanation for the discrepancy in the number of medication errors on the self report and the incident reports could be that not all nurses chose to participate in the study. (KE, p.58)

A final note on when to provide a citation for statistical tests, according to Zeiger (2000): 'For statistical analysis, state the statistical tests that you used and, for tests that are not well known, also give a reference to the report or book that describes the tests as you used them. Well known tests that do not need to be referenced include Student's t test, chi square, standard forms of analysis of variance, linear regression, correlation, and widely used nonparametric tests such as the Wilcoxon signed-rank test' (p.133).

Rigour

It is assumed that rigour will be addressed, whether in its own sub-section or within a broader discussion of the strengths and limits of the methodology.

Ethical considerations

The structure of this section will vary according to the procedures you went through to meet the requirements of your ethics review board (REB), but it typically includes the following (examples from KE are included in parentheses):

- What was sent to participants (e.g., introductory and information letters)
- How it was sent (e.g., with the survey package)
- What it told participants:
  - o study purpose
  - o assurance of anonymity and confidentiality
  - o potential benefits and risks
  - o participation is voluntary
  - o contact information
- What constituted consent (e.g., returning the completed survey)
- What board[s] approved the research proposal; include the approvals in appendices and reference them here. (In KE's case, there are four appendices: approvals plus extension approvals from two REBs.)
- Discussion of the potential risks and benefits for the participants and how risks were addressed

METHODOLOGY AND ANALYSIS IN QUALITATIVE RESEARCH

Although there are major differences in methodology and analysis between quantitative and qualitative research, the decisions you need to make as a writer are very similar. The central argument being made overall and at every point is the same: here is what I chose to do and why, and here is how I addressed any potential problems, both proactively and as they arose.

The organization of MRV's Methodology chapter (which is lengthy, at 58 pages) is included here because it represents a thorough breakdown of a grounded theory process. Notice that the chapter has an overview and summary. Notice too how carefully the headings in the Methodology section suggest an argument from general to specific, moving from grounded theory to constructive grounded theory.

CHAPTER 3 METHODOLOGY AND METHODS

3.1 Overview

3.2 Methodology

   3.2.1 Grounded theory

   3.2.2 Contribution of grounded theory in the 'second moment of qualitative research'

   3.2.3 Constructive grounded theory

   3.2.4 Adaptation and application of constructive grounded theory

3.3 Study design

   3.3.1 Setting

   3.3.2 Sampling strategy

   3.3.3 Inclusion and Exclusion criteria

   3.3.4 Recruitment

   3.3.5 Ethical Considerations

3.4 Fieldwork

   3.4.1 Focus groups

   3.4.2 Interview process

3.5 Transcription

   3.5.1 Stage 1: Making a raw data transcript

   3.5.2 Stage 2: Making the transcripts readable and analysable

3.6 Data analysis

   3.6.1 Constructing initial codes

   3.6.2 Constructing themes, sub-categories and categories

   3.6.3 Constructing the core category

   3.6.4 Memo writing

3.7 Summary

(MRV, pp.5–6)

WRITING UP THE RESULTS OF QUANTITATIVE RESEARCH

The purpose of the Results chapter[s] is to present the results of the data collection and analysis but not to comment on their meaning – that is the function of the Discussion. Researchers often decide, however, to combine their results and discussion; this is especially common in qualitative studies where the analysis and its meaning are intimately connected; in most quantitative studies, however, they are separated for the sake of clarity – the result is presented neutrally until a judgement is made based on it in the discussion which follows. It is important here to distinguish between data, results (or findings) and conclusions.

Data are the facts (from experiments) and text (from interviews) obtained through data collection. For example, the Mean (SD) change in mean arterial pressure in FWM's guided imagery group was 1.58 mmHg (7.63). (Typically, the data are presented in table form in quantitative studies.) A **result** or finding interprets the data, for example,

> There was a statistically significant difference between groups in changes in mean arterial pressure (MAP)(t = 2.36, p = .02); mean arterial pressure increased significantly more between baseline and the last week of available data in the Quiet Rest group (M = 5.93 mmHg, SD = 6.55) than in the Guided Imagery intervention group (M = 1.58, SD = 7.63). (FWM, p.82)

Finally, a **conclusion** gives the implications of the data, for example, that use of guided imagery can improve mean arterial pressure in hypertensive pregnant women.

The chapter often begins by repeating the research question[s] and is subdivided into sections corresponding to the variables studied. Where there are multiple research questions each with a complex set of results, it is not uncommon to have multiple results chapters.

A few tips:

- If there are results that relate to the study design or extraneous variables, present those first, in order to confirm that the design was effective.
- Report the most important result first and move through secondary results to the least important.
- Closely related results can be discussed together in the same paragraph.
- Begin each paragraph with a sentence that states a result, and follow that with explanatory details. In other words, every sentence should be designed to give a result or contribute to one.
- Remember that qualifiers such as 'good' or 'poor' will seem vague and judgemental without supporting evidence, such as comparison data.

I've mentioned 'important' results, but what about the ones that aren't important? Should they be included in the interests of being thorough? The answer here is that just because you found something does not mean it goes into the chapter. Talking about a minor or irrelevant result is distracting because the reader assumes if it is in there, it must be important and then is confused trying to figure out what's important about it.

What about the findings that contest your conclusions? Should they go in? After all, won't they weaken your case and open doubt in the examiners' minds about awarding you that degree? In fact, the opposite is true – omitting contradictory results is what opens the door to doubt. So do include them, and explain why your other results outweigh them.

What should you do if your results do not satisfactorily answer your research question? The thought might cross your mind to give a result that you expected to find, as opposed to the one you did find. Don't fall into this ethical (and career-destroying) trap. Instead, figure out the cause of the discrepancy, give the true result and explain why this was not what you had expected. This advice comes with a caveat – if the results are so negative that your whole study is in jeopardy, it is time to speak to your supervisor.

The reader should not have to read through an entire paragraph of data before coming to the message about the data. For this reason, results are presented as a combination of visuals (tables and figures) and text. All the relevant data are presented in the visual, and the text draws attention to the crucial data.

TABLES AND FIGURES

The word 'visuals' is used to describe tables and figures. A 'table' is a set of columns (*horizontal 'x' axis*) and rows (*vertical 'y' axis*) that show exact numerical (*quantitative*) data. The word 'figure' refers to all other kinds of visuals: graphs, charts, drawings, maps, photographs, and others. The best source of guidance on the purpose and formatting of tables and figures is the sixth edition of the *Publication Manual of the American Psychological Association* (APA, 2010) and the advice below is either based on or consistent with it.

Some general rules about visuals:

- Keep visuals as simple as is feasible.
- Label all visuals.
- Make reference to visuals within the text; they are intended to complement text, not to replace it.
- Place the visual as close as possible to the point in the text that refers to it, but never interrupt a sentence with a visual.

Readers make certain basic assumptions when they approach a table or figure. They expect that:

- written information follows from left to right and from top to bottom
- information in the centre or foreground is more important than information on the periphery or background
- large or thick elements are more important than small or thin ones
- elements that are similar in size, shape or colour are related to each other.

Tables

Tables allow the researcher to present a large amount of data in a compact space. Tables usually show exact numerical values, although in qualitative research they often consist of text. Don't use a table if you only have a small amount of data to present (i.e., a table with only one or two columns and rows). Simply present the data in the text.

- In the text, you must refer to every table and tell the reader what to look for. Discuss only the table's highlights – if the text duplicates all the information in the table, what was the point of having the table?
- There are several common ways to refer to the tables in text, such as these from FWM:

Table 2 provides an overview of the study groups' baseline characteristics. (p.78)

In any one week, the maximum frequency of noncompliance was two occurrences, as represented in Table 3. (p.81)

The differences in mean arterial pressure change remained statistically significant (Table 6). (p.85)

- Do not refer to 'the table above' or 'the table below' or 'the table on p.16'.
- Although the text always discusses the table, the reader should be able to understand the table without reference to the text.
- Data must be arranged so that their meaning is obvious at a glance and so that entries to be compared are next to each other.
- Identify all abbreviations (except standard statistical abbreviations) and units of measurements, either in a note or as part of the title, as in the example below from FWM (see Table 9.1).
- The *APA Manual* (2010, p.127) recommends numbering all tables with Arabic numerals in the order in which the tables are first mentioned in the text. If the manuscript includes an appendix with tables, identify those tables with capital letters and Arabic numerals. For example, Table A1 is the first table of Appendix A; Table B5 is the fifth table of Appendix B. Note that if there is only one appendix, it is labelled Appendix without a letter, but the tables are still labelled Table A1, Table A2, etc.
- The title goes above the table. Table titles should be as brief as possible, but must be clear and explanatory, as in the example below from FWM (see Table 9.1).
- Provide a heading for every column that identifies the units in the column. Indicate in the heading if you are using a particular measure for the units.
- Use footnotes to explain specific items in a column. Use lowercase superscript letters immediately after the word or number. List the footnotes at the left margin of the table, directly below the data. See the example below from FWM (Table 9.1).
- Give the source of your data below the table if it is not your own. If you have multiple sources and have compiled the information into a table, explain this in text.

Finally, let's look at Table 9.1, taken from FWM's results (p.84). Notice how she uses the most important data from it to advance an argument about the value of the findings.

Figures

'Figure' refers to any method for depicting data in a memorable image of the overall pattern of the data. Unlike a table, which presents exact values, a figure gives the reader a visual representation of relationships among data. To express it simply, everything that isn't a table is called a figure. A Table is always a table, but a Figure can be a graph, chart, drawing, photograph, scatter plot, pie chart, a model in theory development, and so on.

In deciding whether to use a table or a figure, ask yourself if you want to give the reader exact values (a table) or if you want the reader to focus on the relationships among the data (a figure).

It is recommended to use a less visually complex, sans serif typeface (such as Arial) on the figure, and a serif typeface (such as Times Roman) in the figure caption. All elements of a figure must be large enough to be legible, generally not smaller than 8 point and not larger than 14 point.

A figure legend (i.e., a key to symbols used in the figure) should be placed within the borders of the figure.

Table 9.1   Sample results table

Table 5.
Group, baseline mean arterial pressure (MAP) and baseline gestational age in predicting MAP change at the last week of study participation

Variable	β	t	Confidence Interval (95% CI)	p
Model 1				
Group allocation	−.24	1.91	−7.15, .16	.06
MAP at baseline[a]	−.27	2.20	.52, .98	.03
Model 2				
Group allocation	−.19	1.51	−0.90, 6.38	.14
MAP at baseline[a]	−.29	2.39	−.49, −.04	.02
Baseline gestation	.24	2.00	−.001, 0.58	.05

N = 60
[a]MAP = mean arterial pressure
Model 1: $R2$ = .16, $F(2, 59)$ = 5.41, p =.007; Model 2: $R2$ = .21, $F(3, 59)$ = 5.12, p = .003
Although group allocation was not significantly predictive of MAP change in either of these models, interaction analysis was undertaken to explore the extent to which guided imagery effect on mean arterial pressure change was influenced by interactions between group allocation and (1) gestation and (2) baseline MAP. These interactions were then added to form a third model, but did not add appreciably to the ability of the model to predict MAP change, and thus were dropped. Overall, even though group allocation did not reach statistical significance, it is important to note its relative contribution to the second model, based on a beta of −.19.

Source: American Psychological Association (2010) *Publication Manual of the American Psychological Association* (6th ed.). Washington, DC: Author.

Table have titles written across the top. Figures, however, have captions that describe the contents in one or more sentences, and the captions are written below the graphic.

WRITING UP THE RESULTS OF QUALITATIVE RESEARCH: DEVELOPING A VOICE

In Chapter 7, we spoke of the need for QL researchers to capture in language the richness and fluidity of human life and health. As a result, in their methodologies, analyses and writing, these researchers need to be flexible and diverse.

One of my concerns in writing this book is that I might be interpreted to suggest that writing a thesis is simply a matter of following the 'templates' provided in the book's dissertation models and suggestions around language use. This is particularly the case in the sections about writing up quantitative research, where there are so many conventions around language structure and use. But the best thesis writing exhibits a voice that is unique to that writer, and is engaging while being rigorously scientific. Qualitative research offers many more such opportunities than quantitative does. So if you are a creative, reflective type, there's a thesis waiting for you to write it.

Such a voice is JL. Her narrative inquiry thesis not only contains a number of her own poems, which enrich her prose text, but the prose itself has a dynamic rhythm and textured vocabulary. At the same time, there is no doubt she has command of the techniques of rigorous data analysis. She also uses a variety of effective strategies to weave her analysis of her participants with their words. Look for these things as you read this sample paragraph from the first of her three Results chapters. It introduces a section headed 'Plugged in', where JL's language captures the sense of excitement her participant conveyed during their interview:

> [1] Patients are inevitably drawn into the complex interrelationship of the technological because they are the principal person that practitioners and their process of care are focused on. [2] Being "plugged in" is a metaphor that describes a process of becoming part of the complex interrelationship of the technological. [3] [Name] described feeling like the **centre** of attention with the **big** lights above him and **all** the people around him ready for his surgery. He **exclaimed**, "I thought I was a **star** on the operating table." (p.108)

[1] In every paragraph, JL begins with analysis. The body of the paragraph then links the point of analysis to the interviews.

[2] JL introduces a metaphor. A metaphor is a comparison of two things that are not literally the same. The patients are not plugged into a wall socket like faulty microwaves, but, as JL explains a little later (p.110), they became part of the technological in the physical act of having their bodies attached to technological objects.

[3] One of JL's techniques is a sentence paraphrasing the relevant portion of the interview, followed by a short or long quotation. Another technique she frequently uses is to weave quoted words into her paraphrase. Notice how JL's vocabulary choices (in bold) evoke the participant's sense of the importance of the occasion.

DISCUSSION: POSITIONING YOURSELF IN THE FIELD

The function of a Discussion section is to answer the question(s) posed in the Introduction; to explain how the results support the answer; and to explain how the answers fit in with existing knowledge on the topic. The Discussion often begins with the answer to your question, because that answer is the culmination of the thesis. It fulfils the expectations you raised in your Introduction, and which the reader has followed carefully through your Methods and Results.

The body of the Discussion also accounts for the ways in which your findings are similar to and different from previous research. If your work is similar to previous research, and had similar findings, that strengthens both. If it took a different approach and had similar findings, that also strengthens both. But if it took a similar approach and the findings were different, the discrepancies must be explained. If different answers to your question have been proposed, why is your answer more satisfactory?

The Discussion goes through the main findings one by one and describes how they are supported (or not) by the previous research that was discussed in the literature review chapter. Here the value emerges of having evaluated them as strong or weak and more or less relevant to the current study. Based on those evaluations, the Discussion needs to be able to argue that the current study supports the findings of (and is in turn supported by) the strongest, most relevant studies, and that the contradictory evidence lies mainly in the weaker or less relevant studies. If all your support is drawn from the weaker or less relevant studies, while the strongest and most relevant contradict you, you have a problem.

COMBINING RESULTS WITH DISCUSSION

It is more common in quantitative research to separate results and discussion into separate chapters than it is in qualitative research, where they are frequently combined. As you can see from the above example from KE, the result is often summarized before it is discussed anyway, so one could argue that having two separate chapters is a 'waste' of space. On the other hand, the result is merely summarized in this example – in KE's Results chapter, it was outlined thoroughly and its rigour and validity argued for.

THE SPECIAL CASE OF THE PUBLICATION THESIS

This type of thesis can be a way to combine the requirement to write a thesis with the increasingly pressing expectation that PhD candidates will achieve publication of parts of their doctoral research project. Masters level students, only some of whom achieve publication, would therefore not be producing a publication thesis. In the case of a practice-based Masters, however, the body of the thesis may consist of all the documents, guidelines, etc., 'published' within an organization as part of the student's project. The benefit of a publication thesis is that you do not need to write up the same material in two completely different forms (article vs. chapter). The articles that you have successfully published in peer-reviewed academic or professional journals during the course of your research project are reproduced exactly as published in chapters that form the body of the thesis. There is no set number of articles, but three to four is common. It is likely that each article is addressing one of the research questions of the whole study. You don't necessarily have to have published the articles as sole author (e.g., if you are part of your supervisor's research group) but you need to have been the one to do the write-up, as well, of course, as taking the lead role in the research itself.

The chapters that frame the articles, such as Introduction and Discussion, serve a different function from those of the traditional thesis. This is because their various traditional functions are already being fulfilled within the articles that form the body of the thesis. The long narrative arc of the traditional thesis is interrupted by the articles, each of which has its own narrative arc, so the framing chapters are tasked with creating a whole out of a set of parts. They do this by arguing that the articles create a single research project that makes a significant, original contribution.

The actual content of those chapters is variable, depending on what you and your supervisor negotiate together (or, in case of a supervisor who operates on the principle of benign neglect, what you yourself decide is the best approach). You will certainly want to include background to the research project; you may want to include a reflexive element; you may want to describe the publication process. Many decide it is important to include the full literature review from the research proposal, on the rationale that the segments contained within the articles may be insufficient for thesis examiners (no editor will ever allow as much space as the leisurely comprehensive review demands). You are likely to offer a review of your own methodology and theoretical framework. For the chapters that frame the articles on the other side, your Discussion chapter should, at the least, demonstrate that your articles together make a single contribution. The conclusions, limitations, implications, contributions and recommendations within each article will be narrowly focused on a particular research question, so these sections in the final chapter[s] should provide the larger picture.

In a different scenario, a thesis based on publications can be a mechanism for giving academic recognition to a body of already published research publications, whether the research is conducted in a professional or an academic context. This is the case with SM's thesis, which encompasses his eleven articles and one chapter, published between 2003 and 2012. In his case, all the chapters written for his thesis, about 10,000 words or 40 pages, are positioned before the texts of the articles. These new chapters include an introductory section that locates himself, his writing, and his theoretical framework within the broader study of anti-social behaviour; a discussion of the methodology and methods he used over his ten years of research; and a critical review of his publications, grouped into the three social contexts of community, public transport and travel to school. The entire argument of the thesis is summarized in the brief final chapter (Conclusions, pp.35–7), and I have reproduced it here in order to track that argument and the ways SM persuades his examiners to accept that his publications are worthy of a PhD. Throughout, I have bolded the phrasing that advances that argument.

[1] **This thesis needs to justify my claim to a PhD** by **demonstrating** that I have made a significant and original contribution; that I have **demonstrated** a significant quality in my understanding and use of methods; and that my work shows a level of continuity and coherence. **I would suggest that** these three criteria are evident in this thesis, as summarised below.

[2] *A significant and original claim*: **I have located my work** broadly speaking within a social interactionist approach and have utilised this theoretical perspective throughout my research and publications. **I have argued consistently** in my publications that anti-social behaviour brings together a wide range of disparate behaviour under one 'umbrella term'.

[3] In my discussion of this process of categorisation [of behaviour as anti-social], I have **provided an original insight** into the way it is defined in practice … My research and the twelve publications included here have explored interactions within the three distinct social contexts **in a completely original way, demonstrating** the particular factors which are **significant** in each of these contexts as well as making broader links across contexts where relevant.

[4] *Research Methods:* The second element of my justification has been the **quality and extensive nature** of my research methods. I have demonstrated **a strong research base** for my publications, utilising a wide **variety of robust methods**, which have developed in scale, complexity and sophistication over the period of my writing. … [Summary of research methods used in articles]. The thesis **demonstrates too** that I am **able to critically review** these methods, **acknowledging weaknesses whilst defending the overall robustness** of the research techniques … .

[5] *Continuity and Coherence:* The publications which I have submitted for this PhD consist of a **coherent body of work**. … [T]here is the **consistent argument** that anti-social behaviour as a concept needs dismantling and understanding as a continuum of behaviours. … I have chosen to group my publications into the three contexts – **there is no squeezing of articles into arbitrary and inappropriate groupings. It is clear that** the articles fit under these contextual headings and that there are **clear linkages** between the articles within each context and a development from one context to another.

[6] *Continuity of my work:* I have a significant amount of data from the comparative European research and **further publications** will be appearing in the next year. [Description follows of future publications and applications for funding.]

[7] **The justification** I have presented in this thesis for the award of PhD through published works **fully supports my claim** that I have made a **significant, original contribution to academic knowledge** in the area of anti-social behaviour. I have **demonstrated**, through the discussion of methodology and research methods, that I have **a thorough grasp** of research methods, enabling me to engage in the high quality research which underpins these publications. Furthermore, my publications form a **coherent and substantial body of academic work** on anti-social behaviour. Finally, the underpinning research and the publications **demonstrate a clear development** in level of sophistication and complexity.

[1] The first paragraph summarizes the criteria the thesis must meet and introduces the structure of the chapter.

[2] In this first sub-section, the first two sentences summarize the claim the thesis makes.

[3] The rest of the paragraph summarizes its originality and significance.

[4] Here, SM summarizes the Methodological Considerations section of the thesis, in which he had argued the strengths and limitations of the various methodologies he used in his articles. The bolding has been added to highlight the language that economically argues for their overall strength.

[5] It was particularly important for SM to argue that his articles form a single body of work, because they were not published within the research framework of a doctoral programme. The issue would not arise in the same way for a thesis where the publications arise from the traditional single PhD research project. Nonetheless, it is always important to discuss the ways in which the articles do form a single research project.

[6] As in the traditional thesis, it is good to include future plans for research and publication.

[7] The final paragraph summarizes the entire argument in support of the thesis.

CONCLUSIONS AND OTHER FINAL BITS

You may feel by this time that you've reached the final chapter for your sanity, but gather your inner strength and keep your eyes fixed on that light at the end of the tunnel.

In many ways, the final thesis chapter summarizes what has come before – after all, the Discussion has already interpreted the results and probably reflected on how the methodology (and you as a person) determined those results. But it has to be more than that. It needs to answer the reader's unspoken question, 'So what?' As a reader, I want to know what good it does to know your findings. How strongly can I rely on them? What do you want me to do with your research, in future research and practice? How does what you've done relate to my concerns in the real world of healthcare and health systems?

Structurally, the final chapter should offer the following:

- conclusions based on the discussion
- the strengths and limitations of your research methodology (and publications, if relevant)

- the implications of your research and recommendations for future research and/or practice
- final reflections/reflexions
- summary of the original contribution of your research

There is considerable variety in how this final material is organized. It is also common for the conclusions to be stated at the end of the Discussion chapter rather than as the first section of the Conclusion chapter.

Now let's explore some writing strategies for the different elements.

Draw conclusions based on the discussion

The word 'conclusions' can be interpreted in more than one way. It can refer to a conclusion in the sense of a logical process (i.e., I had a question[s] that I studied in these ways, producing these results, from which I now conclude the following answer to my question[s]). Or the word can be interpreted in the sense of a pulling together of all the argumentative strands woven throughout the thesis. The language chosen needs to project a sense of confidence but not arrogance. In other words, the language supports the strength of the thesis while not suggesting it has solved humanity's greatest ills. Phrases such as these are typical ways of demonstrating that confidence:

This study found that …

Additionally I have shown that …

This research demonstrates that …

But there are also ways to temper it (without, of course, suggesting your thesis should be rejected):

Despite some limitations, this study established that …

On this basis, I would suggest that …

Discuss the strengths and limitations of your research (and publications)

The strengths and limitations of the research will already have been considered at relevant points in the Discussion. Here, however, they are summarized.

When you come to the end of the limitations section, that crucially emphatic final position, it's good to remind the reader of the study's strengths. It avoids an overall negative impression, and is an excellent transition to the implications and recommendations that follow. Phrasings such as these make the move economical:

Despite these limitations, this study strongly indicates that …

Although exploratory, this research shows a clear path for future research …

Discuss the implications of your research and make recommendations

Your introduction will have established the newness of your research by identifying the gap in our knowledge you intended to fill. Now that you've filled it, it's time to remind the reader of its newness:

[1] Managers **should familiarise themselves with** the evidence on emotional labour and its relationship with burn-out in nurses since they have an important role to play in creating and maintaining the conditions for effective supervision. Managers **should also be open to** the different forms that nurse supervision takes. Ward nurses reported hand-over times as frequent sources of supervision that are not formally recognised as such. ... [2] [T]hese critical support mechanisms **may be jeopardised** if proposed moves to home-based working and virtual teams (who meet infrequently) are implemented. Managers **should be particularly aware that** nurses who are geographically isolated from other team members may be missing out on vital informal support. [SJM, p.131]

[1] The three recommendations in the paragraph are signalled by parallel verb constructions that all use the modal verb 'should', which signals the idea of obligation or necessity.

[2] The modal verb 'may' signals possibility, in this case a negative consequence of a trend within the system that is at odds with SJM's findings and recommendations.

A note on modal verbs: A special class of verbs is called 'modal verbs', which are a type of auxiliary or 'helping' verb. Auxiliary verbs help complete the form and meaning of main verbs. Modals combine with main verbs to express meanings such as ability, possibility, permission, obligation and necessity. The principal modal verbs are ***can, could, may, might, must, should*** and ***would.*** They are useful in many parts of a thesis, but especially so in the implications and recommendations section, where the ideas of ability and possibility, obligation and necessity are particularly important.

Recommendations for future research can arise both from what the study did accomplish and from the limitations of what it was able to accomplish (in other words, an unfilled or newly revealed gap in our knowledge).

Reflections/reflexions

The strand of reflection that has been part of the thesis narrative also needs some final consideration. Like many writers of qualitative studies, including JL, SJM chooses to end the thesis with a brief final reflection:

6.7   Final reflexive considerations:

My professional and personal backgrounds have undoubtedly shaped this study from its conception through to the final preparation of this thesis. What I offer here is my interpretation of nurses' views, experiences and stories and my interpretation is, in turn, shaped by my own experiences: [quotation from Freshwater, 2002]. Freshwater goes on to suggest that the research process itself might be therapeutic, with the possibility of psychological or spiritual development and transformation. Although this appears to be something of a grand claim, I feel it does represent my personal growth and development as a researcher during the course of my doctoral study. (SJM, p.140)

Summarize the original contribution of your research

You will, of course, have lost no opportunity to mention this throughout the whole chapter but now it should be summarized. When she comes to the actual 'Contribution' section, notice how SJM (in the bolded words) economically uses every sentence to focus on an aspect of what she has contributed. As befits the positioning of the section as the final effort to focus on the positives of the research, there is some qualified language here (such as 'offered', 'believe', 'suggest', 'potential') but overall the tone is firm and positive.

Contribution to knowledge

This study contributes an understanding of age-related complexity from the perspective of mental health nurses who work with older people, as well as contributing insights into the experience of nursing complex older people. In common with other qualitative research, the findings of this study are offered as a starting place that requires further exploration and consideration rather than definitive answers. In addressing the first research question, **the study has identified** features of age-related complexity as constructed by registered nurses, **but beyond this I have also** drawn distinctions and comparisons between frailty and complexity (McGeorge, 2011). **I believe that these differences have important implications for** future policy and research involving older people. (SJM, p.139)

10

DISSEMINATING YOUR WORK: PRESENTATIONS AND CONFERENCES

CONFERENCES AND CAREER ADVANCEMENT

One of the likely results of acquiring a post-graduate degree is that your professional colleagues will increasingly call on you to make presentations. Luckily, post-graduate studies give you ample opportunity to practise and hone your skills, and to receive feedback from experts (your supervisor and other faculty) and peers, especially those who are in cohorts ahead of you. Conferences in particular can be an important professional development tool throughout your career.

The main point of attending a conference is to learn about the most up-to-date research and thinking in the field, while networking with both important leaders and new voices. Your main, ongoing source of knowledge of the field is peer-reviewed journals, but a) the publication process is slow (as we'll see in the next chapter) and b) editors do not publish research in progress. Conferences, on the other hand, allow people to introduce and get feedback on their research and thinking while they are developing it. There is also, of course, the chance to holiday in exotic locales, and indeed, the setting of a conference is an important part of the decision to go to it. If you have heavy family and financial obligations, for example, you may seek out conferences in your own geographical area. Or you may be in a position to use conferences as a way to broaden your horizons and travel. Conference organizers are well aware of the adage about 'location, location, location' and will try to generate interest that way. Travel can be very expensive, though (even when you save money with multi-stop flights that drop you off in the middle of the night, or if you share hotel rooms with several other students). Unless you are independently wealthy, speak with your supervisor and/or department before sending in proposals to learn if there is some funding available for post-graduate students to attend conferences.

A note on professional associations and scholarly societies: It is important to join as many of these as you can, as they are excellent for resources and networking, but there are membership costs, and though they are reduced for students, they do add up. Ask around to make sure you join the essential ones. Not least of their benefits are the calls for papers and conference announcements.

A BRIEF GUIDE TO THE ABSTRACT

To apply to present at a conference, you will need to submit an abstract. In fact, throughout your post-graduate career, there will be numerous situations that require an abstract, for example, with funding applications, with articles submitted for publication, and for your thesis. Your abstract will change depending on what the particular situation requires, but the advice below will help in any of them.

What is an abstract?

An abstract is a brief summary, which condenses in itself the argument and all the essential information of a paper, presentation or thesis.

An abstract allows the reader to survey the contents of a document quickly and decide whether to continue reading. It needs to be dense with information but also readable, well-organized, brief and self-contained.

Abstracts are generally 100–250 words, though a thesis or conference abstract may be up to 400 words.

A conference paper may have an audience of a few dozen; the audience for a journal paper may be hundreds to thousands. An abstract, though, has a life of its own in electronic databases around the world. Like a title, it is used by abstracting and information services to index and retrieve articles. Thus, for every person who hears or reads a paper, hundreds may read the abstract.

An abstract competes for attention in a global ocean of literature – it's worth spending some quality time on writing it.

What goes into an abstract?

For a **research paper**, an abstract typically answers these questions:

Purpose:	What is the nature of your topic/study and why did you do it?
Methods:	What did you do, and how?
Results:	What were your most important findings?
Conclusions:	What can you logically conclude through analysis of your data?
Relevance:	How do your findings relate to the theory or practice of your field, or to future research? Do you have any recommendations?

For a **methods paper**, an abstract typically answers these questions:

Name:	What is the name or category of the method, intervention, or tool? If this is an improved version of an existing method, say so.
Purpose:	What is the major reason for developing this method? State the purpose in the form 'for doing X' or 'to do X'.
Features:	What are its key features, how does it work, or both?
Relevance:	Why is this method needed?
Tests:	How was it tested?
Evaluation:	How well did it work?

Tips on writing an abstract

1. Write the abstract last
2. Follow any guidelines you've been given
3. Be accurate
4. Be self-contained
5. Be clear, concise and specific
6. Emphasize points in proportion to the emphasis they receive in the paper
7. Use signals
8. Select key indexing terms

Tip no.1: write the abstract last

Ideally, an abstract should be written as the final stage of an otherwise complete paper. Otherwise it will tend to be vague and/or incomplete. You'll hesitate to be too specific, because you don't know yet what your conclusions will be. You'll start writing uninformative sentences like these:

- ✗ Preliminary results are presented.
- ✗ Policy implications are discussed.

The abstract can be written last in the case of articles for publication, or when you are applying to a conference to present research you have already conducted. On the other hand, this is often not possible in the case of a conference abstract where you may be submitting six months or longer before the actual conference, and may genuinely not know where things will be at that time. Similarly, for a research proposal submitted to a funding agency, you are usually asking for money in order to proceed with the plan outlined in the abstract.

Tip no.2: follow any guidelines you've been given

There are no rules for the exact format of an abstract. However, if the abstract is being submitted to a conference, journal, grant agency, or is part of a thesis or dissertation, the organization or department may issue guidelines for abstracts.

If so, be sure to follow them precisely. Do not try to 'improve' on their format, or think it doesn't matter if you make minor changes (or even major ones!). Differences from an expected format interrupt the reader's ability to concentrate on the text. When your reader has dozens (or hundreds) of abstracts to choose from, this sort of negative attention does not help your case for acceptance.

Tip no.3: be accurate

Make sure the abstract does the following:

- it uses the same language as the presentation, paper or thesis, especially key words and concepts
- it includes only information that actually appears in the paper
- it correctly reflects the purpose and content of your paper
- for a research report, it states if the study extends or replicates previous research

Tip no.4: be self-contained

You can't ask your reader to go elsewhere for an understanding of what you say in your abstract. Therefore,

- define all acronyms and abbreviations (except standard units of measurement)
- spell out names of tests and drugs (use generic names for drugs)
- define unique terms
- do not include references. An exception is made for sources whose theory, method or measure is being used. For example, 'All participants completed the Movement Imagery Questionnaire (MIQ; Hall, 1983)'.

Tip no.5: be clear, concise and specific

- make each sentence as informative as possible, especially the lead sentence
- include in the abstract only the most important concepts, findings, or implications
- the question and what was done can often be written in one sentence:

To examine the effect of an imagery intervention on imagery use of pregnant women, *we required women (n=30) to listen* to a guided imagery session for one hour during six consecutive weeks.

- avoid sentences that contain no real information (e.g., Policy implications are discussed)
- short sentences are preferable but not required. Avoid clusters of nouns and adjectives – they make your sentence shorter but often compromise clarity:

✗ Our study found significant bipolar disorder interepisodic phase functional morbidity.

✓ Our study found significant functional morbidity in the interepisodic phase of bipolar disorder.

- if you give a P value, also give data (e.g., mean ± SD) and the sample size (n)
- use active voice and personal pronouns for study objectives

✗ First, new clinical criteria were attempted to be defined.

✓ I first sought to define new clinical criteria.

- conserve characters:
  - use digits for numbers unless the number begins a sentence
  - abbreviate whenever possible (e.g., *vs.* for *versus*)
  - give per cent change rather than exact data when possible
- don't waste space by repeating the title
- don't waste space with promises – an abstract should deliver:

✗ This study will examine pain control at Hospital X.

✓ Of the caregivers at Hospital A, 53% actively encouraged epidurals for patients who were 'hostile or extremely resistant' to artificial pain control.

Tip no.6: emphasize points in proportion to the emphasis they receive in the paper

- If your paper is a proposal, with fairly equal sections devoted to background, literature review, and your proposed method, those should be the proportions in the abstract.

- If you are reporting on research, the amount of space devoted to results should reflect their importance and level of complexity.

Tip no.7: use signals

a) Signal the parts of your abstract with conventional phrases such as these:

Your question:	We asked whether X inhibits Y …
	We hypothesized that X inhibits Y …
Your method:	To answer this question, we used …
	To test the hypothesis that …, we conducted two trials …
Your results:	We found that …
Your analysis:	Descriptive statistics were used to analyze …
Your answer:	We conclude that X inhibits Y …
	Therefore, …
Your implications:	We suggest that X may play a role …
Your recommendations:	We recommend that X be administered …

b) Choose verbs that signal the parts of the abstract:

- use present tense for the topic/problem/question
- use past tense to describe your method, results and analysis
- use a cautious present tense for implications (*may mediate, can improve*) and recommendations (*should be administered*)
- use simple future tense in a proposal (*I will measure …; This exploratory study will investigate …*)

c) Use transitional words and phrases that signal logical relationships:

Addition:	In addition, also, moreover, as well as
Contrast:	However, nonetheless, although, but, unlike
Comparison:	Similarly, compared with, equally
Causality:	Therefore, thus, consequently, as a result, in conclusion

Tip no.8: [for publications] select key indexing terms

- Choose key words and phrases that will make your paper readily and accurately searchable in databases
- Select terms you would use to find your own paper
- Select current terms, such as medical subject headings (MeSH), that name important topics in your paper
- If necessary, include an indexing term even if the term does not appear in the paper.

SOURCES

American Psychological Association (2010) *Publication Manual of the American Psychological Association* (6th edn). Washington, DC: Author.

Hewitt, J.L. (2001) 'Abstract checklist'. Unpublished instructional material prepared for use at Rice University Houston, Tx.

Landes, K.K. (1991) 'A scrutiny of the abstract, II', in W.R. Hansen, *Suggestions to Authors of the reports of the United States Geological Survey* (7th edn). U.S. Government Printing Office.

Silyn-Roberts, H. (2000) *Writing for Science and Engineering: Papers, presentations and reports.* Oxford: Butterworth-Heinemann.

Zeiger, M. (2000) *Essentials of Writing Biomedical Research Papers* (2nd edn). New York: McGraw-Hill.

EFFECTIVE PRESENTATIONS

Any presentation, especially at a conference, is a summary of the most important information you decide your audience needs to know about your larger topic. The content and organization vary according to the topic and your purpose in presenting it. You may be presenting at the literature review stage, or when you have developed a theoretical framework. You may want to present on methodological issues, or deliver some of your results. The important point is that you will not be trying to compress your entire research project into a single 15- or 20-minute paper or poster. Because a presentation is a summary, you always know much more about the topic than you can include (which is an advantage when it comes to answering audience questions). This means making careful choices about what to include or leave out based on how much time you have and what single message you want to deliver to your audience.

Presentations always contain a verbal element and a visual element, but the proportions vary. For example, a conference paper is a talk supported by PowerPoint slides. A poster is a visual presentation supported by a short explanatory talk, often to a panel of judges.

Like any other piece of writing, a presentation has an introduction, a body, and a conclusion. But it doesn't get written in the same iterative way described in Chapter 3; instead, it is written as an outline of points, major and supporting, that are then fleshed out with evidence and comment as needed.

Visual supports

Visual supports help you to reinforce key points in your presentation and provide supporting evidence and illustrations. The most traditional and simplest visual supports are chalkboards, dry-erase boards, and flip-chart pads, all of which you write or draw on as you present. We don't cover them here, as there is little to say beyond making sure your writing is large, clear, and dark enough to be seen from anywhere in the room.

PowerPoint presentation software allows you to prepare a multi-media slide display that can include text slides, sound and video clips, illustrations and photos. A more traditional form of slide presentation uses overhead transparencies and a projector. Transparencies are not as versatile as PowerPoint but have the advantage that you can write on them as you talk. But we begin with posters.

Poster design

Size: There are no rules for the exact size of a poster, but if you are given specific guidelines for dimensions, make sure you follow them carefully.

Materials: Poster boards are available in standard sizes at office supply stores. Software is available that allows you to design and print your poster as a single sheet, or you can use your computer's standard word processor to produce a series of letter-sized sheets (8 1/2″ x 11″ or A4) and affix them as panels to the poster board.

Layout: There are no rules for exact layout of a poster, but you should choose an overall layout that suggests an arrangement of communication areas. Some common options are:

- Top-to-bottom, left-to-right flow of information in vertical columns.
- Two fields in contrast.
- A centred set of images or data (tables and figures) flanked with columns of text.
- A centred set of images, data or text circled by text or visual blocks.

Leave sufficient white space to create distinct communication areas. Test this by standing back from your poster far enough that you can't read the text – do the white areas clearly define blocks of text and image?

- Label figures and tables clearly and descriptively.
- Use large typeface. The following point sizes are recommended:

Title: 96

Subtitle: 24 point to 36 point

18 point for text

1. Don't use more than two fonts throughout. Also, don't mix serif and sans serif fonts (serif fonts have the little lines on the ends of the strokes that make up the letters; sans serif fonts don't):

Times New Roman 14pt   Arial 14pt

2. Be creative, but don't overdo the formatting to the extent that it obscures the information.
3. DO NOT WRITE ALL IN CAPITALS. IT IS IRRITATING.

Poster writing style

You need to maximize the limited space on a poster by writing in a style that is dense with information. This section will show you some ways to minimize the number of linking words in your sentences in favour of substance words. Keep in mind, though, that your writing also needs to be crystal clear to the reader, and balancing density with clarity isn't always easy. A poster has to be self-contained:

- define all acronyms and abbreviations (except standard units of measurement);
- define unique or unusual terms the first time you use them.

Save space wherever possible: use digits for numbers unless the number begins a sentence. Abbreviate whenever possible, such as 'vs.' for' versus' or 'e.g.' instead of 'for example'.

You can also compress your sentences by using lists and 'gapping', a technique in which all non-essential words are removed. Here is an example from a Nursing student poster:

Search criteria

Key words used: needle exchange programme (NEP), HIV, AIDS, statistics, mortality rates, cost of treatment.

Sources searched: WHO, Centre for Disease (CDC), National Institute for Health and Clinical Excellence (NICE), charitable organization websites (e.g., UNAIDS).

Dates searched: 1995–2010.

Why this range?

- NEPS not in operation in the UK until 1985
- 1995–2010 represents the most up-to-date information

Visual elements of posters

The visual elements on a poster can include tables, figures (defined below), and any formatting elements that help to highlight the different sections of the poster. In general, try to keep the formatting elements as simple as possible. Too much detail and variety confuses and distracts the viewer from getting the message about what is most important.

As with text, where we signal importance through position and length, we have a number of ways to signal the relative importance of visual elements. Viewers expect information in the foreground to be more important than information in the background or on the periphery. They expect large visuals to be more important than small ones. They also expect things with the same size, shape, location or colour to be related to each other. Take advantage of this in designing your own layout.

Tables: Tables are used to display a body of related data so we can easily see changes and make comparisons. Make sure you refer to your tables within the text and explain why you are including them. The title of the table (always located *above* the table) needs to be clearly descriptive of the message of the table.

Figures: Anything that isn't a table is classified as a figure. Here are some of the most common types and what we use them for:

Photograph or drawing	To show what something looks like
Map	To show where something is located
Diagram	To show how something is put together
Line graph	To show the relationships between two or more sets of data plotted on a grid created by horizontal and vertical axes
Bar graph	Like a line graph, these plot a series of values on two axes, but using bars instead of points joined by a line. Each bar represents a quantity of something. Used to compare quantities and show trends
Flow chart	To show the sequence of steps in a process
Organizational chart	To show the vertical and horizontal structures of an organization
Pie chart	To show proportions and percentages

Presenting your poster

You will want to seek out opportunities to do a poster presentation at research days and conferences. Typically, at such an event, a large room is given over to posters, which are arranged in a number of long rows. The organizers will set up ranks of poster stands, to which each participant affixes his or her poster. A panel of expert judges will make its way up and down the rows, examining the posters, listening to the participants' descriptions of their posters and asking questions. At the end of the day, the best poster presentation will be awarded a prize. Here are some tips for presenting to the judges:

- Talk to the judges, not the poster. Face them and turn to the poster only to point to specific items you want them to focus on.
- Use verbal cues to direct their focus (e.g., 'If you look at the results of the pilot smoking cessation programme [point at figure], you'll notice that …').
- Look around at your audience and make eye contact. Don't stare ahead of you, at the floor, or at your poster.
- Speak clearly, loudly, and slowly – the acoustics in poster rooms are rarely favourable. They tend to have low ceilings in proportion to their length and width, and they can get very noisy at well-attended events.

It is also important to do the following:

- Arrive early and spend as much time as possible near your poster. One of the benefits of research days is the opportunity to meet new people – don't waste the opportunity by wandering away after the judges have been by.
- Be ready to expand on the poster contents. As the day progresses, your audience constantly changes. Some viewers are only mildly interested; others want to learn all about your research. You should prepare several versions of your remarks, from 30 seconds to 5 minutes.
- NETWORKING: Be ready to exchange contact information with interested viewers.
- Be ready to respond to both praise and criticism graciously.

POWERPOINT

PowerPoint design

PowerPoint software and others like it allow you to create digital slides which you project through an LCD projector and control through a computer. The basic structure is as follows:

Title slide: title of your presentation, your name and affiliation
Overview slide: point form outline of what you will be presenting
Introductory slides:

- background on your topic
- why the topic is important
- previous approaches
- your approach

Body
Concluding slides:

- clear statement of the overall message of your presentation
- a look ahead
- acknowledgements
- consider designing an interesting final slide that can remain on-screen while you take questions, such as a photo representing your topic.

PowerPoint slides should be visually interesting but not overwhelming:

- Use bulleted points and parallel constructions [test 1 … test 2 … test 3].
- Use an Arial font, at least 16 point, **bolded.**
- For tables and figures, make sure the reproduction is clear and large enough to read. It is easiest to read tables in black text on a very light background. Include only one complex or two simple tables/figures per slide.
- Don't overcrowd but do fill the frame – no tiny objects in the middle of an empty screen.
- Don't overdo multiple colours and whizzing objects.
- Viewers with colour blindness will be disadvantaged if you use two colours based on the same primary colour (e.g., pink lettering on a red background, orange on yellow, or green on blue).

PowerPoint presentations

Some wag once noted that the big advance of PowerPoint is that it lets the audience sleep in the dark. Don't let that be your presentation!

Keep the introduction short. Tell your audience clearly and concisely what you are going to cover, and then get right into things while they (and you) are at their freshest. 'Taking command' in this way also helps you psychologically to get past any nervousness you've been feeling.

Focus on the critical points. You can amplify during the question period.

Use wording that establishes a hierarchy of importance, as well as numerical listings: 'The most important factor in the recent rise in TB cases has been … Two other factors that have had an impact are, first, … and second …'.

As you come to specialized terminology, define any terms you believe will not be known to your audience.

Announce your graphics, and if the content of the slides is not self-explanatory, explain it.

Don't be the presenter who flips through slides without a word of explanation, sublime in the misconception that what is crystal clear to her or himself will be equally clear to the audience. On the other hand, don't be the presenter who laboriously reads every word of text on the slides and elaborates on each number and image. Instead, train yourself to engage with your slides when necessary but not otherwise: in your speaking notes, highlight the points at which you will turn briefly to the slide and gesture, using words (preferably not a laser pointer) to direct the viewers' attention. Indicate both location (e.g., 'the table on the right gives values for …') and meaning (e.g., 'in this video clip we see a typical client interaction').

Always end at the end. That is, if you're running out of time, skip to the end. If you've rehearsed properly, this shouldn't happen but sometimes the unexpected surprises us – problems with equipment, for example, or a programme day that is running behind time.

DON'T FORGET TO BREATHE: USEFUL TIPS ON ORAL PRESENTATION

Some presenters write a paper and read their presentation verbatim from the prepared text (or even recite it from memory). I attended one session where the presenter also handed round copies of the text so we could read along – it was the longest 30 minutes of my life. Presenters use these strategies because they fear they will freeze up in front of an audience. They worry about being asked a question and not knowing – or not remembering – the answer. But unless you are a very fine actor, you will find it surprisingly difficult to deliver a prepared text with the fluidity of natural speech and you risk quickly losing the interest of your audience.

A better strategy is to write up a detailed outline that includes both paragraphs and bullet points and to train yourself – through as much rehearsal as you can possibly squeeze in – to speak from that instead of a fully prepared text. It isn't difficult to build a presentation outline:

- Use one side of the page only and number every page clearly. Leave a great deal of white space.
- Make headings larger and bolder.
- Lay out your points and supporting evidence using a combination of short paragraphs and multilevel bulleted points.
- Underline key words or ideas you will want to emphasize.
- As you practise speaking from your outline, mark cues on the text for pauses. Pauses create emphasis. They also help you remember to breathe!
- Mark cues for referring to your slides.

Use these principles to guide you in structuring speaking notes and deciding what to include:

1.   The introduction should (if necessary) introduce yourself. Then say why you are making this presentation (e.g., to report on an existing programme or intervention; to argue for a new programme or intervention); outline what the presentation will cover; and give any background or definitions the audience will need.

2.   The body of your talk should be clearly divided into sections that each present a single major point with arguments and/ or visuals to support it. The amount of space and time given to individual sections should reflect their importance in relation to your overall purpose and topic. If your purpose is to present a review of the literature on the topic of pain management interventions for neonates, your largest section will be devoted to a summary and evaluation of the research literature, subdivided into the different categories or strengths of research evidence. Is your purpose to propose a new agency in a priority neighbourhood? – you will want to give the most space to identifying the issues in the neighbourhood and how this particular initiative will address them.

3.   The conclusion should summarize the content and main argument of the presentation. The final section usually gives recommendations for research, theory, and/or practice. End with a brief list of acknowledgements (two or three individuals or organizations that assisted you with information, funding, or technical/research support).

4.   The audience at a presentation is not a passive entity. The individuals who make it up will be responding to your performance and it will show in their faces and body language. You can train yourself to make use of this. Many presenters find it helpful, as they come up to face the audience and begin to speak, to focus on the friendly, interested faces – especially their friends. As time goes on, it will be easier to observe the audience as you speak and make occasional eye contact. As you proceed, you will feel an overall sense emanating from the room: interest and enjoyment, or perhaps (but hopefully not!) boredom and confusion.

5.   The audience will also engage actively with you through questions and discussion at the end of your presentation. In some presentation settings, such as a seminar, questions and discussion will take place at points throughout, as well as at the end. If you are in a large room or auditorium, when someone asks a question, repeat it loudly and clearly – many in the audience will not have heard it. Doing so also gives your brain time to organize your answer.

6.   Think of presenting as a type of theatre. You are there not just to inform but to do so in a way that engages – even entertains – your audience.

'Locating' your presentation

•   What is the physical space like in terms of size, shape, seating, lighting? Where are you standing within that space? Imagine how different it would be to present in these two common presentation settings:

- A classroom or seminar room with seating for 20–25 around a long, rectangular table. You stand at the head of the table and don't need a microphone. There is some light in the room even when darkened for PowerPoint, which is projected onto a small screen on the wall. Or you may present using a poster and/or flip chart, which everyone can see easily. You can make eye contact easily and observe the audience's reactions to what you say. You can also move around the room if you need to.
- An auditorium with seating for 100–200. The presentation area is at the bottom of a pit and the seating is raked (i.e., rows of seats rise at an angle so much of audience looks down at you). The presentation area is lit; the rest of the auditorium is darkened so you cannot see anyone clearly. You stand behind a fixed lectern in a corner beside the screen and speak into a microphone attached to the lectern. Your presentation is projected onto a large screen behind you.

- What are the acoustics like in the room? Acoustical quality is determined by a number of factors: the shape and dimensions of the room, the height of the ceiling, the materials used to build the room, the number and arrangement of people and furniture, and where you stand within the room.
- How good is the lighting? Are you in a room with windows letting in natural light that must be blocked so a screen can be used for PowerPoint? Is it an inner room with artificial lighting? Is the room uniformly lit or can portions of it be darkened (which allows slides to be seen while the audience has light to make notes by)? Or is the presentation area lit while the audience is in darkness, as in a theatre?
- What equipment is available to you and how good is the quality? Is technical support available to help you set up or in case of equipment problems?
- If you will be using a microphone, what kind is it? Is it fixed to a podium or lectern (you have no mobility)?; is it a 'stem' microphone that cradles on top of a stand and can be removed and held in your hand (you can choose whether to stand still or move around, but you lose use of one hand to do so)? Is it a microphone that you clip onto your clothing with a battery pack that clips onto your belt or waistband (you have complete mobility)? Or is the whole presentation area wired for sound (complete mobility)?
- When you are using a microphone, speak at your normal volume. If you hear popping or a screeching noise, lower your voice or stand back a little. If you are not using a microphone, pause a few seconds into your presentation to ask those at the back of the room if they can hear you.
- Where will you be standing in the room? Will you be behind a lectern or free to move around? The ideal position is where the audience can see you and the screen at the same time, you don't block anyone's view, and you can easily operate a projector or computer.
- Is it a space you are well acquainted with? If not, can you gain access ahead of time to familiarize yourself?

Preparing to deliver

You cannot rehearse too much or too often, and you should practise with a focus on developing three areas: clear, fluid delivery of your talk; a comfortable stage presence; and facility with using the technology of your visual supports.

- Rehearse, rehearse, rehearse. Spend extra time on the introduction, as this is the part where nervousness is most likely to make you stumble.
- Time yourself.
- Try to rehearse in a setting that approximates where you will be presenting or, if you can't, imagine yourself in such a space. Stand in the position you will occupy in the room.
- Ask a colleague, friend or family member to watch you rehearse. Ask them if you have any nervous gestures or recurring speech patterns that distract them from what you are saying, or are even annoying. Do you sway from side to side or back and forth? Do you fidget with your clothing or jewellery? Ask them to ask you questions at the end – every person who rehearses with you will have some different questions and some that will be the same, which will give you some idea of what you are most likely to be asked. The questions they ask will sometimes surprise you, things you hadn't thought of – and now you're prepared for them.
- Make sure you learn how to operate any technology you'll be using and rehearse with it until it becomes a seamless part of your talk.
- Make up a list of questions you might be asked. Imagine an audience in front of you. Imagine them asking you the questions. Answer out loud as if they were there.
- Practise safe redundancy – bring backup copies of your presentation using a different technology. For example, you can bring a PowerPoint presentation on both a notebook computer and a USB key. You can also email it to yourself ahead of time and retrieve the presentation directly into an on-site system in case your own computer fails to connect with the system.
- Bring whatever physical aids you might need, for example, throat lozenges, tissues, and a recyclable/reusable bottle of water.
- Get plenty of sleep.
- Avoid caffeine, but do hydrate well with water.
- Dress professionally. Understand that your audience is not just judging your presentation – they are looking to see what kind of professional you are becoming. But also dress comfortably – now is not the time for new shoes. Even if they are comfortable, their newness is a distraction.
- Hold nothing in your hands except your notes. Should you use a laser pointer? On the one hand, they are obviously useful for directing the audience's attention. On the other hand, nothing conveys nervous energy more than a twitchy red dot jiggling across the screen. Many presenters prefer to use hand gestures and language instead: 'The mortality rates in the middle column of this table ... '. If you have bolded the important information in the table, your audience will have no trouble locating it.

- Don't bury your hands in your pockets or clutch a lectern.
- Don't worry if you feel nervous. That just makes you more nervous. It is natural to experience stage fright and many experienced presenters still feel twinges before they 'go on'. In the vast majority of cases the things we fear – freezing up, making some disastrous error, the audience hating our talk, etc. – never happen and the nervousness itself fades very quickly once we start. As well, the more rehearsing you have done, the more secure you will feel. It also helps to make a conscious effort to breathe and relax. Relaxation is cumulative – as you learn to do it, it gets easier until it becomes a habit. Here are a couple of relaxation exercises to get you started:
    - Drop your hands to your sides; let them hang inert, dead weight; let them feel so heavy you don't think you can lift them. Do this any time you can, such as on public transport, or relaxing at night. When you've got good at relaxing your hands, move on to learning to relax your shoulders and neck. Shoulders and neck tend to be the spots where nervous tension collects first.
    - Practise breathing, something you can do anywhere at any time. Become deeply aware of the fact that you are breathing – feel your lungs rise and fall as if a tide is coming in and out. Relax your throat and feel the air rushing through. Open your mouth and throat wide as if in a yawn (it's even better if you can make yourself yawn). Keep that openness and relaxed feeling as you exhale. Be so open and relaxed that you can make air come through both mouth and nose at the same time. Track the air down to the base of your lungs – feel your belly fill out and your ribs strain against your back muscles.

How to perform

These tips are based on the voice training that singers and actors receive to help them achieve a comfortable stage presence and a clear, strong delivery. Mental exercises reduce nervousness and increase confidence. Physical exercises provide stamina and increase the volume and clarity of your voice.

- Here is an exercise to relax you for the start of your talk. It will also oxygenate you and strengthen your speaking voice: In the minute before you go on, become aware of your breathing, in and out slowly, as deeply as is comfortable. Once you are standing in position, take a few seconds for a last comfortable breath, let it out, and take a normal intake. Hold your head high and look around the room as you begin to speak.
- Some people feel 'safer' if they stand close to a fixed object such as a lectern or console, perhaps touching the object occasionally to help with the sense of being grounded. Other people are more comfortable if they can move about the presentation area and gesture freely (but not excessively) with their arms and hands. In this way, we all have our own comfort levels, as long as we avoid the extremes of rigidity and wild movement.

- Begin S-L-O-W-L-Y: You will naturally speed up as you speak, especially if you are nervous. The slowness may sound awkward to you, but to the audience you will seem deliberate and confident.
- Speak to the whole room. Make eye contact.
- Project your voice to the back of the room or auditorium: in other words, lift your chin so that your throat is extended but not uncomfortably so. Look to the back of the room and, as you speak, imagine waves of sound travelling in a high arc right to the back row of seats. This psychological exercise will have a physiological effect, helping your voice to travel for a longer distance.
- Don't swallow your consonants: North Americans especially can be guilty of lengthening their vowels and sliding over consonants, often running words together or dropping final consonants altogether. The overall effect is that the audience can miss important words, or need to strain to understand what you are saying. A good exercise in rehearsal is to overemphasize final consonants to the point that they sound overly noticeable to you. If you listen carefully to actors on television or movies, you will notice that they 'overpronounce' their final consonants in this way.
- Don't let your good habits fall away as you near the end of your talk – before starting your conclusion, pause, take a comfortable breath, and articulate clearly as you signal the coming end. Use phrases such as 'In summary, ...' or 'To conclude with some recommendations,...' .
- Body movements can work either for or against you. Fidgeting nervously with jewellery or tugging on clothing will distract your audience from your presentation. On the other hand, gesturing with your hands at the same time as you emphasize key words creates interest and facilitates understanding. Turning your head so you end up looking at every section of the audience instead of facing rigidly ahead allows you to face every member of your audience and include them all. Do this even if the lighting in the room is directed towards you so that you can't actually see the audience. After all, the audience doesn't know you can't see them.

Notes for multilingual speakers

Many post-graduate students whose first language is not English, and who have not yet learned to be proficient in the language, lack confidence in their ability to lead a discussion and respond to questions. They often worry about not understanding what others say or ask, or they worry that others won't understand them accurately. They find it challenging to understand the idiomatic speech of the native speakers in their courses, or the array of global accents among their colleagues in today's multicultural university and healthcare settings.

Many English language learners worry that, under time pressure to respond to questions, they won't find the words to express their ideas clearly and are concerned about making grammar mistakes. Or they worry because they need time to think of answers in their first language and mentally translate into English. (One of the strategies of successful English learners is to spend a few minutes each night thinking *in English* about what happened to them that day, or repeating out loud in English things they have learned or read.)

A few tips:

- Don't be afraid to ask people to clarify what they've asked (e.g., 'I'm not sure I caught your meaning'), especially if they've used some idiomatic expression or made some cultural reference you don't know. You will find people are generally happy to explain.
- Don't feel you need to answer quickly. Take a few seconds to think through your response. The audience isn't going anywhere; they will wait.
- Don't feel you need to speak quickly. Slow speech sounds deliberate and thoughtful, and also allows the audience time to absorb what you are saying.

Group presentations

This chapter has consistently spoken as though you are presenting alone, but you may be asked to make a collaborative presentation in which you present as a member of a group. Group presentations differ because they add a social dimension.

Your goal is to maximize the contributions of each participant while minimizing the possibility of interpersonal conflicts. A clear planning process will smooth your path.

In your first meeting, explore how much knowledge and what kind of knowledge each person brings to the group (e.g., one individual is a very strong writer/editor; another has clinical experience with the topic; a third works well with multimedia). At the same meeting, decide on a timeline and schedule of meetings. Also, decide on specific roles for each member, such as editor or facilitator (the person who coordinates what individual members are doing and checks on their progress). One individual should record all this and circulate it afterward to the group, so there is no confusion (or contention) later on about when and what everyone is to do.

A frequent question is whether it is better for each person to work independently on separate sections and to send their material, after an agreed-on period of time, to the selected editor of the group for melding into a single piece. We could call this the 'All-to-one' method (Collins and Bosley, 1995). Often the poor editor must then go chasing the inevitable one (or more!) who fails to send the work on time, or who has done a bad job, or done the wrong job. Another problem is that pieces written separately by individuals with different writing styles don't always meld easily. The editor may end up having to do a major rewrite, which may not sit well with the original writer and adds unfairly to the editor's workload.

Another editing pattern is the 'All-to-All' strategy, where the group works collaboratively from start to finish, sitting together for lengthy research, writing and editing sessions. Composition by committee, as it were. Unfortunately, interpersonal conflicts can quickly arise. Writing by committee is also time-intensive, hard to schedule, and doesn't necessarily produce good writing.

So, to sum up the problems, collaborative work is time-consuming, hard to schedule, and can lead to conflict. On the other hand, leaving everyone on their own for too long can result in widely disparate pieces that don't connect in topic or style.

Two other editing patterns identified by Collins and Bosley (1995) are worth considering instead: the 'One-to-One-to-One' pattern, in which one member drafts a part and passes it to a second, who edits and passes it to a third, etc. Everyone edits, but the final person should be the 'senior editor' who can evaluate and incorporate the best feedback and put all the sections together. Finally, there is the 'All-to-One-to-One' pattern, where everyone writes individual parts and the editing is split between a content editor and a grammar/style editor. This is my personal preference.

When it comes to preparing for the oral presentation, each member should practise on her or his own, but it is wise to schedule at least two group rehearsals. Rehearse using your visuals, ideally in the space where you will be presenting. If you are all going to take part in the presentation, set firm time limits for each person and enforce them during group rehearsals. One of the best lessons I ever learned was from one professor who came to our first seminar class equipped with an egg timer. He overturned it at the start of the first student's presentation, and cut the student off with a curt 'Thank you, that will be all' the instant the sand finished running through. At the second seminar class, we were all finishing on time.

It is important to establish a harmonious atmosphere when you are working in a group. Given the stresses each member experiences balancing school and personal demands, tempers can flare and small disagreements can be become turf wars and personal disputes. Be polite, listen respectfully and carefully to the other participants' ideas. Try to seek agreement rather than dwell on differences of opinion. Be willing to compromise – a group working together can produce more and better results than the sum of the work individuals would produce.

FOR FURTHER READING

Collins, C.E. and Bosley, D.S. (1995) *Technical Communication at Work*. Fort Worth, TX: Harcourt Brace College.

Quitman Troyka, L. and Hesse, D. (2007) *Simon & Schuster Quick Access Reference for Writers* (3rd Canadian edn). Toronto: Pearson/Prentice Hall.

11

DISSEMINATING KNOWLEDGE THROUGH PUBLICATION

INTRODUCTION

Frequent, high-quality publication has become essential to a successful research career. As McAlpine and Amundsen (2011) point out, 'globalization and emerging digital network technologies have fundamentally altered the context and practices of academic communication (Starke-Meyerring 2005), raising the bar for success by requiring a higher rate of research productivity and increasingly the demonstration that research has an impact internationally' (p.7).

SOURCE

McAlpine, L. and Amundsen, C. (2011) 'To be or not to be?: The challenges of learning academic work', in L. McAlpine and C. Amundsen, C. (eds) *Doctoral Education: Resesarch-based strategies for doctoral students, supervisors and administrators* (pp.1–13). Dordrecht: Springer.

Why publish?

The narrow answer is because your supervisors say they expect it of you; in other words, publication has become expected within doctoral programmes (and often encouraged at the Masters level). However, the research community you are joining publishes for a variety of broader and more important reasons: to advance knowledge, to advance their careers, to inform the field, to educate the general public, to warn of risks, and/or to challenge current perceptions and practices.

Journal and book editors will not accept any piece for publication that does not advance knowledge and understanding in some way. (This is one of the factors that make it more difficult to publish research at the Masters level where, unlike doctoral research, an original contribution is not a requirement.) For example, a piece might contribute a new way of thinking about an existing problem or it might introduce a new problem; it might give details about an already developed system; or it might make a theoretical advance, a clinical advance (e.g., an intervention), or an improved methodology (such as an assessment tool).

When to publish?

Should you be trying to publish as soon as possible, in other words, as soon as you have enough data collected to support an article? Or should you wait until you have written chapters of your thesis and then adapt them into article form? This is an issue that requires serious discussion with your supervisor early in your programme. On the one hand, supervisors have a vested interest in prompt publication by their students – it advances their own careers. You yourself may be eager for publication, in which case your interests meet. But you also have an interest in a quick degree completion, and publishing while writing the thesis does slow you down. Talk this over with your supervisor and decide when (or if, in the case of a Masters) is the best time to undertake publication.

What to publish?

Broadly speaking, journal articles and book chapters will either try to tell an entire story or will offer a piece of a larger puzzle that the author[s] are working on. Because of its greater length, a book chapter is more likely to focus on some bigger picture, within the theme of the book. The space restrictions of journals tend to dictate the puzzle approach, so that the totality of someone's research emerges over time as it develops and grow.

A mistake frequently made by new authors is trying to tell their entire research story at once, or the opposite – choosing a part of it that is too limited to interest anyone. It's a good strategy to use the journals you are interested in as models. First, see what they say in their submissions guidelines about the type, length and scope of the articles they seek. Analyze the scope of the articles themselves – how large is the territory they cover? Then be realistic about your choices for your own article.

Who is the audience?

In considering what and where to publish, it's crucial to consider who you want to reach. Are you targeting the researchers and academics in your field? A wider, multidisciplinary audience? Clinicians and other professionals? The general public or perhaps a segment of it?

Authorship

The majority of articles in scholarly and professional publications, as your own readings will have shown you, are co-authored. This reflects the fact that fewer research projects of sufficient complexity to merit publication are carried out by only one person. In addition, researchers welcome the opportunity to collaborate. It is a compliment to be asked to co-author, as it means your colleagues not only value your work but also feel that having your name on the publication is an advantage. A great deal is riding on authorship, as Fine and Kurdek (1993) noted in an early but still fully relevant article on authorship attribution in student–supervisor collaborations:

> In academic settings, decisions regarding promotion, tenure, and salary are heavily influenced not only by the number of publications in peer reviewed journals but also by the number of first-authored publications (Costa and Gatz, 1992). Similarly, in applied settings, professionals with strong publication records are often considered to have more competence and expertise than their less published counterparts. (p.1141)

Fine and Kurdek argue that two types of ethical dilemma can arise in these authorship decisions. First is when the supervisor takes authorship credit that was earned by the student. The second arises when the student is given undeserved authorship credit. In this case, the supervisor's motive may be to promote the student's career, but it falsely represents the student as more expert than she or he actually is, and gives an unfair advantage professionally (p.1143).

SOURCE

Fine, M.A. and Kurdek, L.A. (1993) 'Reflections on determining authorship credit and authorship order on faculty-student collaborations', *American Psychologist*, 48(11): 1141–47.

As a graduate student, your supervisor may ask you to contribute to an article he or she is working on with other authors, or you may be writing an article yourself based on your thesis research. Even in this situation, it is often the case that your supervisor will be a co-author, both to increase the chance of acceptance and to reflect their role in your professional development.

Authorship decisions (perhaps negotiations is a better word) can be delicate. And perhaps nowhere else in the supervisory relationship are the unequal power relations revealed so clearly, because students have the least amount of say in the decision.

On what basis should the decisions about authorship be made? To be considered an author, each person should contribute substantively to the design and conduct of the research, and to the writing of the article. The general rule is that the name of the principal contributor should appear first, with subsequent names in order of decreasing contribution. As the Vancouver style guidelines specify, 'acquisition of funding, the collection of data, or general supervision of the research group, by themselves, do not justify authorship' (*Uniform requirements for manuscripts submitted to biomedical journals*, available at http://epe.lac-bac.gc.ca/100/201/300/cdn_medical_association/publications/mwc/uniform.htm). The caveat is necessary because all too often authorship, or even lead authorship, is given for one of these reasons, when really all it entitles the person to is an acknowledgement. To avoid this, and for other reasons to do with ethics, journals commonly ask authors to describe what each contributed.

Conflict around authorship sometimes arises in cases of supervisor–student collaboration. The student may feel that she or he 'did all the work' of data collection, analysis and write-up (this is, after all, related to their thesis research) and so is entitled to first authorship. The supervisor, on the other hand, may feel that the student needed extensive supervision, or perhaps additional analyses were required that were beyond the scope of the student's current abilities and training. As the *APA Manual* notes, it may be necessary to revisit initial decisions on authorship if this turns out to be case (APA, 2010, p.18).

In a worst-case scenario, it may simply be the practice of a supervisor to take first authorship for all their students' articles, on the grounds that this is the work of 'their' research group. This is more common in medical sciences than in nursing sciences. Supervisors whose main concern is to establish their students in their burgeoning careers will be generous in giving first authorship to the student, as long as they feel that it is appropriate.

THE PUBLICATION PROCESS

Choosing a journal

You are less likely to go trolling for books to publish in than journals, because book chapters are frequently by invitation or by special call. In considering journals, ask yourself:

- Who are the primary readers of this publication? Will my article contain information that is new and of current interest to this group?
- What is the nature and quality of the articles in the publication?
- For what purpose is this publication intended? Am I in agreement, or at least comfortable, with it?

Also consider the status of the journal within the profession. The prestige of a journal stems from the material it publishes. Journals publishing sound articles on strategic work conducted by professionals from large, well-known centres attract a wide, international readership. They also receive the most citations. It follows that these journals receive the most submissions of the best articles and have the highest rejection rates. Thus, you risk losing anywhere from weeks to months of valuable time. On the other hand, acceptance is a significant honour and reflects well in your CV. So, once you've identified a potential journal, balance the following factors to make your choice:

- its level of prestige
- the nature and breadth of its readership
- its accessibility through commonly used indices
- the likelihood of your article gaining acceptance

Table 11.1   Speciality vs. multidisciplinary journals

	Speciality journals	Multidisciplinary journals
Examples	*Pain*: 'Provides a forum for information about the nature, mechanism and treatment of pain.'	*International Journal of Nursing Studies*: 'Aims to contribute to the advancement of the science and practice of nursing and interrelated disciplines worldwide by the international dissemination of sound information based on rigorous methods of research and scholarship.'
Advantages	1. These journals hit 'your' people 2. You can use more of your field's special language (what sounds like jargon to an outsider), without the need to explain, define or simplify 3. May publish special issues, perhaps opening an opportunity that fits your research well. This also narrows the number of submissions you will compete against compared to a regular issue 4. Offer more room to show all your work and methodology. 5. Room for in-depth discussion	1. Reaches a wide audience 2. High impact factor and prestige 3. Consolidates and expands your thinking 4. May publish special issues
Disadvantages	1. Lower impact factor 2. Sometimes a very narrow audience	1. No room for full work and methodology 2. No room for in-depth discussion 3. Very low acceptance rate

Editorial decision-making	1. Journal may be associated with an academic or professional society
	2. Decision-making:
	  • editor-in-chief
	  • section editor[s]
	3. Reviewers assigned from:
	  • editorial board
	  • outside (sometimes author's suggestion)
		1. Aimed at a wide audience
		2. Must have outstanding importance
		3. Decision-making process:
		  • editorial staff decide whether to send paper for peer-review (most manuscripts declined without outside review)
		  • typically less than 10% acceptance

Impact factors and citations (for better or worse ...)

Calculating a journal's impact factor is a way of evaluating it, presuming to reflect both its impact on the field and its quality. An impact factor is 'a measure of the frequency with which the *average article* in a journal has been cited in a particular year ... calculated by dividing the number of citations in the current year to articles published in the two previous years by the total number of articles published in the two previous years' (Davis, 2004). Individual papers are evaluated based on the number of citations they receive in other publications. Publication in high impact journals and receiving a large number of citations give the benefits of prestige and wide dissemination of your work. These also have career impacts, for example, in terms of awards, fellowships, grants, jobs, and promotions (Davis, 2004). Having said that, impact factors and citations are not universally useful measures as they inherently disadvantage areas of narrowly specialized interest or certain types of research.

Journals themselves will frequently list their impact factor. Information on the most frequently cited, highest impact journals and papers in a field is also available in *ISI Journal Citation Reports* and the *Citation Index*.

Querying an editor

Pre-submission queries are common and can be sent to multiple editors simultaneously. This is an important point because the article itself must NEVER be sent to more than one journal at the same time (more below on this). Queries can be made in-person or by email. Chapter 10 spoke about the importance of conferences for networking, and the opportunity to meet journal editors is one such opportunity. It can be somewhat awkward to introduce the subject of your ambitions to publish in conversation. A line I have found to be very successful is "Do you mind if we talk business for just a moment?' But do speak to them – even buy them a coffee or a pint, if the two of you are so inclined and time permits – and ask about their journal. Are they interested in seeing an article from you? Ask about their upcoming publication schedule. Do they have any special issues planned? These are typically planned at least a year in advance. Make sure you follow up with an email and submission as soon as possible.

Email queries are, of course, much more common. If you are responding to a call for papers from the journal itself, be sure to identify at the beginning of the message what call you are responding to and where you read it. Then briefly describe yourself and mention any previous publications if you have them. Then give the title of your article and a brief description. Finally, ask if they would be interested in seeing the manuscript and thank them for their attention. Use the principle that the reader should be able to see your entire message on one screen. Sign off with your first and last name followed by your institutional signature: full professional name and degrees; position[s] you hold (or 'PhD candidate' if you are a fulltime student); institutional name[s], address[es], and contact information.

The cover letter

If you speak to an editor at a conference and they express interest in seeing a piece from you, follow up as soon as possible. In your cover email, remind them where and when you met, and that they expressed interest in seeing your article. Something like this is typical:

Dear [first name]:

It was a pleasure to meet you at the National Health Conference in Tottenham last week, and I appreciated the interest you expressed in seeing some of my work. As I mentioned, my work on [topic] is a [brief description]. Please find attached [title]. I look forward to hearing from you. Yours truly, … .

In this situation, using the editor's first name is acceptable because you have met and conversed in person. A 'cold' query is formal, typically 'Dear Dr. X'. The journal website will list its editorial board, so don't use a general form of address, such as 'Dear Journal Editor' – it leaves the impression that you are disinterested in them and just casting a broad net of queries.

Submitting the manuscript

On its website, a journal will have a link to its guidelines on content, length and style for authors who wish to submit manuscripts. The word 'guidelines' is misleading – these are not suggestions, they are requirements. Though this is advice given frequently in this book, it always bears repeating: follow the guidelines obsessively. Check and recheck to ensure you do everything they ask. For example, if you have used one style in formatting and citing, such as APA, but the guidelines specify another (e.g., Chicago), take the time to make the changes. If your margins are 1.25 inches (3 cm) and they ask for 1 inch (2.54 cm), make the change. You may not understand why they ask for the things they do, but you don't need to.

 The ethics of submitting for publication are complex, so avoid these career-ending mistakes:

> *Multiple submissions:* You cannot submit the same article to more than one journal at the same time, or to another journal while one is still considering it. If you put an editor through all the work of sending your article out for peer review and deciding to accept it, only to learn from you that some other editor has just picked it up, that editor will never again read anything you send. Worse, your reputation will spread and others will avoid you too. This may seem rather unfair to you in these days of long response times – and indeed you would be right – but you must remember that editors do not deliberately hold you up. The process simply takes time because it involves the input of a number of very busy people.

> *Duplicate publication:* You cannot submit articles to multiple journals that are essentially the same piece with minor revisions – a different introduction and conclusion, perhaps. This is considered a duplicate publication. Also, if a paper you presented at a conference or meeting is being published in the conference proceedings, you cannot also submit it to journals. If it is not being published in proceedings, you can submit it but make sure to tell the editor in your covering letter where it was originally presented. This information will then appear on the first page of the published article. The only time duplicate publication is acceptable is when a paper is reproduced as a chapter of a book.

Padding the CV: Sometimes authors will try to enhance their CV by publishing multiple articles from the same study, splitting the results up so that each article reports on one related set. But unless there is a distinct difference in the message of each paper, simply splitting the same material into multiple pieces is no way to enhance your professional reputation.

Initial screening

Once your submission is received, an editor will assess whether the subject and length are appropriate for the journal; if it 'fits' with the journal's upcoming publication plans; if the article merits publication on the basis of its research, argument, and writing; and if the style follows the submission guidelines. If there is no point to proceeding to peer review, based on this assessment, the editor will return the manuscript with a cover letter explaining the reasons for the decision. Sometimes the letter will leave the door open to resubmission if major revisions are made (if you are unclear whether the letter does in fact leave this open, ask the editor to clarify before you spend a lot of time on revision). If the rejection comes because the article is not suitable for their journal, or not suitable in the foreseeable future (e.g., if they have recently published an article on a similar topic), the editor may recommend other journals you might submit to.

If the article passes the initial screening, you will receive a letter acknowledging receipt and outlining the journal's process for reviewing it, as well as their timeline.

The review process

Peer review means that the journal has a policy of asking experts in the article's topic to evaluate it before accepting it for publication. A clinical journal will also ask a statistician to review your data analysis. Sometimes journals will ask you to suggest reviewers you do or do not recommend to review your work (though you shouldn't offer suggestions uninvited). Why would they ask you and why would you want to make a recommendation? First, because this is your research area, so you can be expected to know the most authoritative voices in it and/or whose feedback you would most value, or who you feel would 'get' your work best. On the other hand, there may be past negative history, either personal or professional, that you feel would bias a particular person's perspective on your work. While this may seem antithetical to the idea of a blind review process, it can help ensure that the most appropriate reviewer is chosen. If you are working in a very narrow field, you may easily guess the identity of your reviewer anyway.

The reviewer will submit two sets of comments to the editor, one for the author and one set of private comments to the editor. To the editor, the reviewer will comment on

- appropriateness to journal
- quality of methodology, results or theory
- technical issues (e.g., if statistical consultation is needed)
- novelty/impact
- rating: accept, accept with minor revision, needs major revision, reject
- willingness to review revision (Davis, 2004)

The editor will then communicate one of the following decisions to the author:

- unqualified acceptance
- acceptance pending specific minor changes
- deferred decision based on a satisfactory revision
- rejection (Bell, 1995, pp.276–9)

A note about rejection

Rejection is emotionally difficult, but remember that all writers receive rejections. There is an apocryphal story about a famous author who, asked to give a talk on how to become a successful writer, came in silence onto the stage carrying a briefcase and a hammer. He pulled a long piece of rope strung with sheets of paper out of the briefcase, and then nailed the ends of the rope to either side of the stage so that it hung like a clothes-line. He then turned to the patiently waiting audience, told them that these were all the rejection letters he'd ever received, and concluded, 'And this is how you become a successful writer'. End of talk.

Whether the story is true or not (and I have heard it attributed to more than one famous author), it makes its point. We all need to learn to deal with rejection and move on until we succeed. It does, though, become easier once you are established in a writing and publishing routine. At that point in your career, you will have multiple projects in various stages along the pipeline, from initial conception to final galleys. The fate of any one piece is diffused when rejection of one may be followed closely by actual publication of another.

Rejection also does not mean the death of an article – it simply means sending it out to a different journal, perhaps after revision if you feel the reviewer's comments warrant it.

Responding to a reviewer's comments

- Remember that the comments are about the paper, not you. When we fear negative response to our hard work, our natural defensiveness kicks in (and trust me, it doesn't necessarily go away with long experience of dealing with reviewers' comments). Anything that isn't outright praise feels like a daggerpoint of criticism and rejection.
- Comments (especially those painful negative ones) are an opportunity to see your work through a new lens and are an important tool for improving both research and writing over the long term.
- Make sure you address every request for change individually in your reply. Cut-and-paste the request at the head of each response. Wherever possible (i.e., don't bother for minor editing changes), begin by thanking the reviewer for making the suggestion (e.g., 'thank you for suggesting more statistical support. This will make the case stronger'). Then detail precisely what you did to respond to the request (e.g., 'I have added a table on p.8 to include statistical data on X'). If you choose not to make a requested change, explain why. It is not helpful to write things like 'I already did what you suggest on a different page. Can't you read?' Instead, consider whether the reviewer might be right – perhaps the information would be clearer to the reader if relocated. Or persuade the reviewer you understand their concern but have a good reason for your decision (e.g., 'I originally considered adding the data at this point but decided to put it on p.xx because …')

Working with an editor

Journal editing is among the many duties that academic researchers undertake (duties which include supervising post-graduate students such as yourself), sometimes by founding and editing 'their' journal, sometimes by taking a turn at the helm of a larger journal. For smaller journals, editors volunteer their time, often in exchange for a temporary reduction in their normal workload, and may be assisted by one or two persons who help with technical aspects of production. At the other end of the spectrum are journals with a staff of professional editors plus technical support. Each editor manages particular aspects of the editorial process and reports to a senior editor who makes the final decisions and oversees production. There may be a large editorial board or individuals who act as section or associate editors. Although you may be dealing with a single 'point of contact' editor, be aware that there are quite a number of people involved in the process of reviewing and publishing your article, all of them busy and often overloaded with work. As a result, patience on your part is a virtue, as is ensuring that you meet all requested deadlines.

Publication times

- Pre-submission inquiries (days–a week)
- First submission (weeks–months)
  - first review (weeks–months)
  - revision (you control this within a time-frame set by the editor)
  - second review (weeks–months)
  - additional revisions and re-reviews
- After acceptance (1–6 months)
- Galleys (weeks)
  - Submit corrections to galleys (you control this within a time-frame set by the editor)
  - Online and print publication (1–6 months) (Davis, 2004)

SOURCES

Bell, L. (1995) *Effective Writing: A guide for health professionals*. Toronto: Copp-Clark.

Davis, K.D. (2004) 'Publishing your work in scientific journals' [PowerPoint presentation], 9 Dec. Toronto: University of Toronto, Faculty of Medicine, Institute for Medical Sciences.

Huth, E.J. (1990) *How to Write and Publish Papers in the Medical Sciences* (2nd edn). Baltimore: Williams & Wilkins.

12

PULLING INTO THE STATION: FINAL TASKS

OVERVIEW

- Out of the tunnel but not in the station … the final elements
- Checking for mechanical consistency
- Submitting the thesis
- The viva/defense

OUT OF THE TUNNEL BUT NOT IN THE STATION … THE FINAL ELEMENTS

You have finished the final chapter and perhaps the adrenaline is fading fast, but unfortunately, though you are out of the tunnel, you are not yet sliding into the station. There are a number of final elements that complete the thesis manuscript, and a great deal of attention to detail is needed. They are discussed here in the usual order they appear in the manuscript:

Title page

- Remember that your title is the first thing the reader sees. Try to read it through their eyes. How clearly does it describe your study?
- The most common form for academic titles is to have a main title, a colon, and then a subtitle. You'll notice that three of our six models do this; see p.4. Notice, though, that the other three do not, and this is perfectly fine.
- To format the title page, follow your institutional guidelines to the last comma or space.

Abstract

You will find advice on writing abstracts on pp.127–132

Acknowledgements

You may be feeling eternal gratitude to your supervisor and committee, or you may be counting the days until they are out of your life. But in the latter case, if you are tempted not to acknowledge them, remember that they may not be entirely out of your life. As your career moves forward, you may well cross paths with them again. It is always wise to thank them. Certainly if you have had a supportive and collegial relationship with your supervisor and committee, you should feel free to praise them in some detail for the specific ways they have mentored and helped you develop as a scholar and researcher. It is a rare supervisor who will not drink in the words.

It is also important to acknowledge financial, material and technical supports, as well as the people you worked with in your study site[s]. Specialized supports such as librarians and statisticians or the writing centre are often included. And of course, you will not want to forget a thank you to your participants. Most people also use this section to thank family and friends for all their support during your years of study. They have sacrificed for your degree, too, whether in emotional or physical supports. How you decide to 'speak' to them in the acknowledgements is always a personal choice, and there is no right or wrong except in the context of your relationship. Some of us are subtle and circumspect in the ways we address family and good friends in the public arena of publication; some of us are fulsome and detailed.

Dedication

Some people include a separate dedication page; others feel they have expressed all the thanks they wished to in the acknowledgements.

After wrestling with all the conventions and expectations, unspoken or otherwise, of thesis writing, this page is your reward. You may dedicate this thesis and all the hard work and accomplishment it represents to whomever you choose. To a higher power, if you are spiritually oriented. To the love of your life or your life's partner (hopefully they are one and the same). To parents, best friends, a mentor, your kindergarten teacher … You may choose to be formal and brief ('With love to …', 'In memory of …') or to wax poetic. It's up to you!

Table of contents

If you took the advice in Chapter 4 (p.40) to use the table of contents as an organizing tool right from the inception of your research project, your table of contents is already complete because you have been updating it as you've written the proposal and thesis. The only task left now is to check for consistency. Print out the table of contents and check off each line as you go through the thesis.

There is no set format for a table of contents. Here are some variations you could use:

CHAPTER 1: TITLE OF CHAPTER

Title of Section

   Title of first sub-section

   Title of second sub-section

Title of Next Section

Alternatively, you may choose to use a stepwise progression of numerals:

Chapter 1: Title of Chapter

   1.1 Title of Section

      1.1.1 Title of first sub-section

      1.1.2 Title of second sub-section

   1.2 Title of Next Section

There are other variations, such as not indenting at all.

Lists of

- Tables
- Figures
- Abbreviations
- Appendices (spelled Appendixes in APA Style)

Glossary (also called List of Terms)

If you feel that your thesis contains a great deal of specialized terminology that you have needed to define in the text, you may decide to include a glossary that brings all the definitions together into an alphabetized list.

Thesis chapters

References

Appendices and other supplemental material

Appendices function to show the examiners that you did the right things at every stage of your research. Appendices include examples of the raw materials of your study: information and consent letters, ethical approval[s], instructions to participants, your data collection instruments and measurement tools, and perhaps samples of items completed by respondents, such as surveys.

Make sure that appendices are numbered or lettered (APA Style uses letters: Appendix A, Appendix B, etc.), and that they appear in the order in which the text mentions them. In other words, the text should not begin by mentioning Appendix C. Print out your list of appendices and go through the text to check off each one as you come to it, and re-label them if necessary to reflect their actual order in the text. If you are using APA Style, note that it has a peculiarity: the normal way of pluralizing an English word derived from Greek, such as 'appendix', is by changing the 'x' to a 'c' (appendices); APA Style, however, pluralizes the word as 'appendixes'. (The same is true for 'index' and 'indices/indexes'.)

CHECKING FOR MECHANICAL CONSISTENCY

By this I mean ensuring that minor details of spelling, punctuation and formatting are identical throughout the entire thesis. If you don't and one of your examiners turns out to be a 'grammar cop' (and there seems always to be one), she or he will have a wonderful time slashing and burning through your thesis. There are a number of things to watch out for, and it is a good strategy to go through the thesis multiple times, each time concentrating on one. This is not to say you should ignore others as you encounter them, but just circle them in order to find them easily later on – don't pause to correct them now. Instead, keep focused on your mission for that particular read-through. Here are some major things to look out for:

> *Spelling:* Canadians face a particular challenge in spelling consistency. Sitting culturally (and linguistically) between the British and the Americans, they always need to decide whether to use '-our' or '-or' endings (e.g., behavior/behaviour), and whether to spell certain verbs with an 's' or a 'z' (e.g., analyse/analyze). Whichever you decide on, make sure you are consistent. If you quote from an author who uses the opposite, do not change theirs.

> *Hyphenation:* Do you vary among 'health care', 'healthcare' and 'health-care' somewhat randomly? All are acceptable but you need to choose one. Similarly, establish in your own mind whether you will, in general, choose to use hyphens or not, for example, 'population based' or 'population-based'.

> *Formatting and headings of tables and figures:* The more similar your formatting of tables and figures, the clearer they will be to the reader, for example, if the titles or column heads of three tables are identical except for one key term that changes. As another example, the same note may be needed under a number of tables or figures. It takes a sharp eye to make sure that all the elements that are repeated across some or many visuals are identical. Even if they started out that way (which requires an attention to detail that is difficult in the drafting process), a change made to one visual is not always carried over to the others. Slowly the consistency starts to drift.

Headings

Formatting of headings and subheadings needs to be consistent throughout. If you choose to use APA Style for your heading levels, check that you have used the following five top-down levels of heading:

1: Centered, Boldface, Uppercase and Lowercase

2: Flush Left, Boldface, Uppercase and Lowercase

> **3: Indented, boldface, lowercase paragraph heading ending with a period.**

> ***4: Indented, boldface, italicized, lowercase paragraph heading ending with a period.*** Text of the paragraph starts after the period

> *5: Indented, italicized, lowercase paragraph heading ending with a period.* Text of the paragraph starts after the period

(APA, 2010, p.62)

SOURCE

American Psychological Association (2010) *Publication Manual of the American Psychological Association* (6th edn). Washington, DC: Author.

There are many variants, however. Using all uppercase for CHAPTER TITLES is very common. Whatever levels of heading you use, make sure every chapter is the same. Your table of contents can act as your checklist.

Formatting decisions

Maintaining consistency in formatting is an area that is surprisingly challenging. This category includes your choices about typeface (such as italic, bold, underline) and font size (which should generally be 12pt. Times Roman, but some like to use a larger font such as 14pt. for headings, and fonts as small as 8pt. are used for notes in tables and figures). Margins should always be 1" (2.54cm) all round. My solution to the problem of remembering how I have decided to handle these decisions is to maintain a file called 'Formatting'. Once I've decided, for example, to use single quotation marks rather than italics to highlight the names of important theoretical concepts, I note that in the file. The note is much easier to find and follow than to constantly be searching for examples in my text.

SUBMITTING THE THESIS

You might think this would be a one-line section: Hit the send button.

But sometimes even smart and organized people get tripped up at this very late stage. It is easy, in the obsession of writing when you feel you're trapped at the bottom of a black hole, to think that everything else will just take care of itself. But with this philosophy, you could emerge from the black hole to discover that you've missed a deadline or omitted a crucial step in assembling or contacting your examiners. I speak from sad experience. One of my examiners approached me to ask if we could move my defense date back just a few days so that he could attend a conference, for which he graciously offered to sponsor me. I made the naïve assumption that, as a committee member, he would never advise me to do something to my disadvantage. It was only when it was too late that I realized I would now miss the deadline for convocating that term by two days. I would have to pay tuition for an additional term, no small sum of money for the privilege of sitting idle for several more months. There was no ill will on the part of the examiner – he simply assumed that I would be tracking my own responsibilities, and he was right to make the assumption. Luckily for me, my supervisor (perhaps feeling a little guilty at not having watched me more closely) was willing to argue all the way up to the office of the university provost to get me an extension.

The message here is never to underestimate the power of bureaucracy and other people's calendars to throw a wrench into things at the last minute. As the expression goes, paranoids live longer. As you approach the point of submission, it is ever more important to be in regular touch with your supervisor, your committee, and your department or other relevant offices.

THE VIVA/DEFENSE

A typical viva (in the UK/Australia) or defense (in North America) begins with the candidate waiting outside a room while the committee discusses preliminary thoughts on your work and decides on the details of how the defense will proceed. Then comes your presentation itself (as brief as 20 minutes or as long as 60–90 minutes) and questions from each examiner, perhaps in more than one round (often another 60–90 minutes). You then retire to pace the corridor while the examiners deliberate.

The North American term 'defense' is perhaps an unfortunate name for the final rite of passage in the thesis process. It suggests armed adversaries lying in wait to ambush you, reveal all your deficiencies as a researcher and human being, and deny you the degree you've spent years working for. The UK/Australian term 'viva' (for 'viva voce', living voice) provides a more reassuring picture of a newly fledged member of the community expressing her or his voice. In reality, while the defense often results in requests for minor revision and occasionally for major ones, it is rare for a candidate to be denied their degree at this stage. Think of it from your supervisor's point of view – her or his career is judged partly on an ability to foster the new generation of researchers. If there were serious issues with your research, how likely is it that your supervisor would have let them stand unaddressed?

In the vast majority of cases, the defense functions more as an exit seminar, a scholarly discussion rather than a rigorous examination. The committee (or the external in Australia, where oral defences are uncommon) sees itself as a gate-keeper, ensuring your work makes a well-researched contribution, but also as the openers of the gate, ready to welcome you into the community. How you experience the defense is also influenced by how you see yourself coming into it, whether you feel you are a novice researcher taking the first step in a career, or an already experienced researcher seeking validation from peers.

Why, then, if the result is overwhelmingly positive, can the prospect of the defense be so nerve-wracking? Here are a couple of possible reasons:

1. You may have lingering memories of the defenses you've gone through during the course of the programme – defending your proposal, comprehensive oral exams – when the examiners would indeed have turfed you out if they felt it was warranted.

2. Academic history is rife with tales of disastrous defenses and near-misses. I myself recall with a chill the half-hour, or half-eternity as it seemed, waiting in the corridor while my committee convinced one of the externals to cast a vote in favour of acceptance. Though vastly outnumbered by the number of successes, these are the stories that survive and are retold. There have been externals who dramatically uncover a fatal and basic flaw in the research, such as in regard to a key variable or assumption. Petre and Rugg (2004) recount the story of a candidate who spent years producing research on mushrooms that showed a startling new cycle in their growth pattern, but omitted to account for the fact that the central heating in the mushroom sheds went on and off at those exact intervals. Or an examiner might reveal a flaw in an assumption lying behind the research. Here Petre and Rugg tell the very amusing (though not to the candidate) story of a safety helmet designed to absorb shock without causing brain damage, based on the

design of the woodpecker's beak, without considering that perhaps woodpeckers do sustain brain damage (p.194).

3.   But let's focus on the likeliest scenario – the viva/defense as a scholarly discussion in which you have a number of points you want to be sure you make. One candidate summarized this very well in a pre-defense interview with Chen (2011):

They will be taking a look at how well I communicate what's in the thesis. So I have already submitted the thesis and I think that it's been approved. So I think at this point they are really looking at how well I understand it, how well I can communicate these findings, and I think that basically they want to clear up any concerns they might have about what I wrote. They want to see how well I understand my own project, and they are looking to see how well I communicate and disseminate those findings. (p.107)

First, though, let's talk about preparing for the defense. There is a good deal of traditional advice available, and it is traditionally given because it works:

- Get as much information as you can from your supervisor, other faculty, candidates who have already defended, and the university website. Attend workshops if they are offered by the university.
- Seek information not just on the nature of the defense but also on the examiners. This will be much easier, of course, if you were involved in selecting them in the first place, as you will already have done background research on them. Seek out their publications. What is their theoretical approach? What methodologies does their research use? By understanding their individual expertise and the lens through which they view research, you can better predict their response to and questions about your own work.
- At many North American universities, especially in the US, defense presentations are open to all members of the department or faculty, and are advertised in notices posted in paper and online. If this is the case, take every opportunity to attend and take note of at least these things:
  o   The candidate's presentation style, both PowerPoint and oral. In two columns, you can make notes on what you think would work for you and what you would want to avoid.
  o   The kinds of questions the examiners are asking, especially examiners who are also on your committee. It is difficult to think outside the box of your own knowledge of your thesis when you make a list of possible questions, and hearing examiners may give you new insights into what they might also ask you.
- As soon as you know where the defense will be held, go in to evaluate the physical space and technology. Rehearse there as many times as you can.
- Try to organize a small group of colleagues and stage a mock defense, where you present to them as your 'examiners'. They too will one day

defend, so there is a benefit to them of figuring out how the minds of examiners work. Include your supervisor if possible. Some departments require supervisors to organize mock defenses.

- Make up a list of possible questions – see some samples below.
- Re-read your thesis, perhaps simply to review its details, perhaps trying to see it through an examiner's eyes.
- Follow all the other presentation advice on pp.132–144.

Having a list of possible questions is a good idea, but you cannot expect that examiners will necessarily ask exactly the questions you have listed. A better approach might be to divide your questions into categories, and be prepared, when the real questions come, to slot them into their relevant categories rather than make comparisons with the actual questions you'd prepared. I think that Chen's (2011) list of categories, adapted slightly here, is very helpful. You'll notice that they mirror the actual chronological process of deciding on a research topic, through the research process, and towards the future:

1. Motivation: why and how did you decide on this topic?
2. Location: what in your personal experience and expertise led you to this research area and helped you conduct it (or limited your ability to conduct it)?
3. Contribution: what is the contribution of your work to theory, research and/or practice?
4. Theoretical framework: why did you use this particular framework? How did you develop your theoretical constructs? What is the contribution of the framework as you developed it?
5. Literature review: how did you choose these types of literature to review? Why didn't you choose other areas? Why did you (or did you not) look at particular authors? Why did you interpret their work a particular way?
6. Research design and methodology: What led you to choose various individual aspects of your design, participants, setting, instruments, analytical tools, etc.? Would you do anything differently if you could? How might that have changed your findings?
7. Generalizability/Implications: What implications do your findings have for researchers, policy-makers, practitioners, administrators, or other relevant groups?
8. Limitations: what do you see as the problems in your study? What limitations do they put on its contribution? How would you correct them in future studies?
9. Further work: what more could you do with your data? How would you follow-up on the work in this thesis? What aspects of your work could be taken further, and how?
10. After your degree: what are you going to do after you get this degree? How do you plan to disseminate your work and/or put it into practice? (Chen, 2011, p.103)

Chen (2011, p.105) also offers another way of considering the questions examiners might pose, derived from Trafford's (2003) analysis of 25 UK doctorate defenses in various disciplines: Group A (technical questions about the dissertation structure and content);

Group B (literature-based questions); Group C (questions about research practice); and Group D (conceptual questions about theory, findings, conclusions; contributions to knowledge; and disseminating findings).

After the presentation and questions/discussion are complete, you retire to allow the examiners to deliberate. If your supervisor emerges after an eternity with a frown, it is likely a sign the committee has recommended major revision that might even require a new defense. But – far more likely – if your supervisor emerges after an eternity with a smile on her or his face, you are brought back in to be congratulated and told your thesis is accepted, with or without some revision. One of Chen's (2011) participants captured the excitement and promise for the future that this moment reflects, and so it is perhaps fitting to end this book with her words:

> They were so welcoming to me afterward… . I can't believe how amazing that experience was. We had sherry up in the Chair's office, and they took pictures, and they hugged me. I thought [I was] very welcomed as a colleague. So it completely changed how I feel as a researcher, because … it felt a little bit like I was being welcomed as a researcher … Like, I passed and now I am a colleague. (p.108).

SOURCES

Chen, S. (2011) 'Making sense of the doctoral dissertation defense: a student-experience-based perspective', in L. McAlpine and C. Amundsen (eds) *Doctoral Education: Research-based strategies for doctoral students, supervisors and administrators* (pp.97–114). Dordrecht, The Netherlands: Springer.

Petre, M and Rugg, G. (2011) *The Unwritten Rules of PhD Research* (2nd edn). Maidenhead: McGraw-Hill/Open UP Study Skills.

Trafford, V. (2003) Questions in doctoral vivas: views from the inside. *Quality Assurance in Education*, 11(2), 114–122.

INDEX